THE HEALING ENERGIES OF TREES

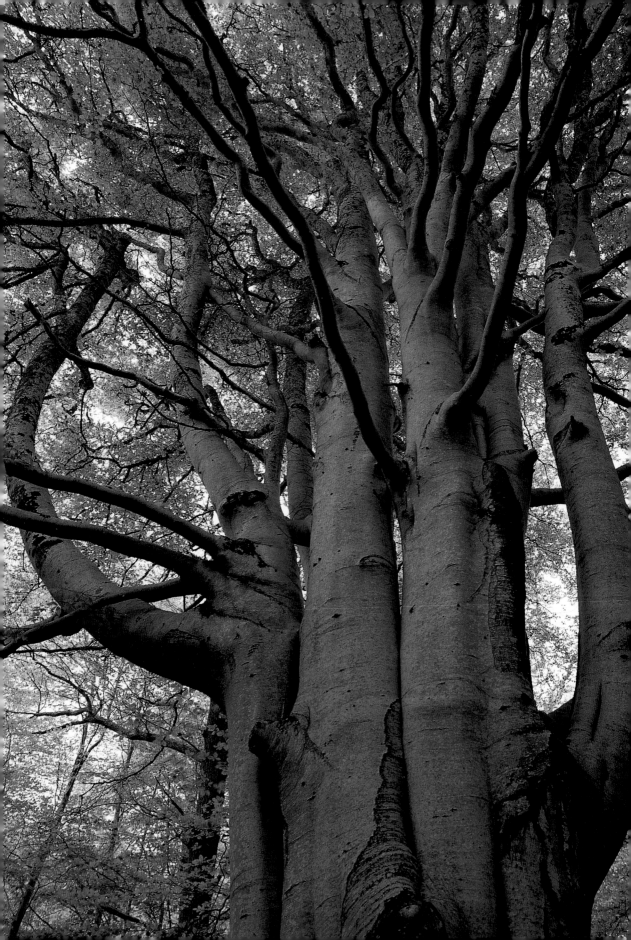

PATRICE BOUCHARDON

THE HEALING
ENERGIES OF
TREES

JOURNEY EDITIONS

Boston - Tokyo

First published in the United States in 1999 by Journey Editions, an imprint of Periplus Editions (HK) Ltd., with editorial offices at 153 Milk Street, Boston, Massachusetts 02109.

DISCLAIMER
The author of this book is not a physician, and the ideas, procedures, and suggestions in this book are intended to supplement, not replace, the medical and legal advice of trained professionals.

All matters regarding your health require medical supervision. Consult your medical practitioner before adopting the suggestions in this book, as well as about any condition that may require diagnosis or medical attention.

The author and publisher of this book are not responsible in any manner whatsoever for any injury that may occur directly or indirectly from use of this book.

ISBN: 1-885203-71-3

Library of Congress Catalog Card Number: 98-87315

Distributed by

USA
Charles E. Tuttle Co., Inc.
RR 1 Box 231-5
North Clarendon,
VT 05759
Tel: (802) 773-8930
Tel: (800) 526-2778

Japan
Tuttle Shokai Ltd.
1-21-13, Seki
Tama-ku, Kawasaki-shi
Kanagawa-ken 214, Japan
Tel: (044) 833-0225
Fax: (044) 822-0413

Southeast Asia
Berkeley Books Pte. Ltd.
5 Little Road #08-01
Singapore 536983
Tel: (65) 280-3320
Fax: (65) 280-6290

Canada
Raincoast Books
8680 Cambie Street
Vancouver, V6P 6M9
Tel: (604) 323-7100
Fax: (604) 323-2600

First edition
05 04 03 02 01 00 99   10 9 8 7 6 5 4 3 2 1
Design by Lucy Guenot
Cover design by Jeannet Leendertse
Printed by Printer Trento Srl, Italy

To Sylvie, Nils, and Iona

AUTHOR'S ACKNOWLEDGEMENTS
As I finish writing this book, my thoughts
turn to all the people who have taken part in
my various workshops. What I most want to
thank them for is that sparkle in their eyes
when they have made a leap of understanding
that touches the soul. Each of these is a
wordless encouragement for me, for nothing
motivates me more than to see someone
waking up to who they really are.

I would like to thank all the people who
take part in this adventure and who work
with so much devotion and generosity to
organize my seminars; in particular Monique
Fonjallaz, Lieve Bonne, and Heidi and
Francis Girardet who welcomed me to their
practice and encouraged my skills as a therapist. Special thanks are due to Lieve for the
stimulus, and the surprises she often springs
on me, in asking me to take my work further.

For this, my first book, I feel I have been
very fortunate to meet the Gaia team.
Working with them has been an enriching
experience, and even though there have been
a few upheavals, they have always maintained
their respect and understanding. Thank you
to Eleanor Lines who had the idea of contacting me and helped sketch out the main lines
of the book. Thank you to Pip Morgan for
breathing new life into the project through
his intelligent and sensitive understanding of
what I wanted to put across. Thank you to
Katherine Pate for her help in developing a
clear structure for the book and for her edit-
ing which has respected my ideas. Thank you
to Lucy Guenot for her sense of harmony and
of what is beautiful, and for her understanding of the subject (apart from the spiral of
consciousness!). And thank you to all the staff
of Gaia Books Ltd, whose professionalism has
contributed to the quality of this book and
will contribute to its success.

To produce a book in a language that is
not one's native tongue demands the kind of
help that Helen Caradon has provided. Apart
from her talent in translation I would like to
thank her for her commitment, which has
meant being ready to work hard whenever
needed. Her views and comments on the
book have often been very valuable.

Contents

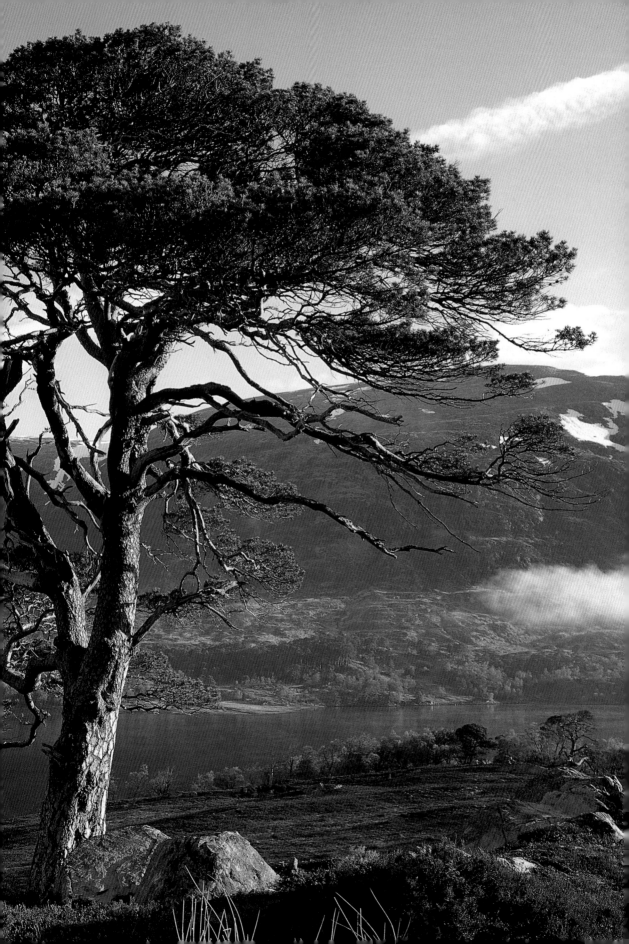

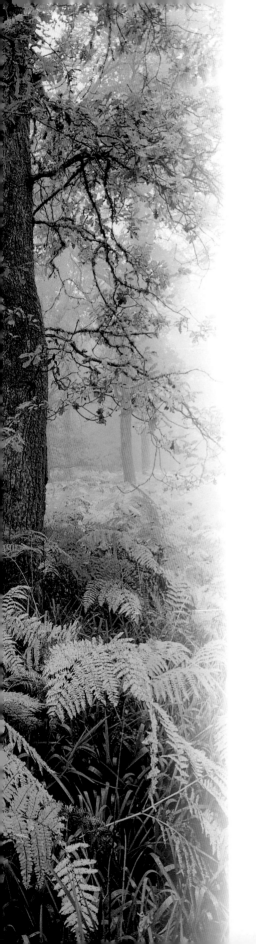

Introduction

From my earliest years I have been drawn to trees. As a child, when I looked at trees they would sometimes hold my gaze a long time, often prompting a kind of waking dream. Beyond their strength and their beauty was a mystery that drew me and touched me deeply. I wanted to make the acquaintance of the trees. It seemed obvious to me that an exchange with them was possible, that there was a doorway which would give access to a veritable kingdom. But I couldn't find a teacher who understood what it was that I wanted to learn, and so my interest in trees evaporated.

Many years later my wife Sylvie and I were asked to run a farm for four months while the owners were on holiday. In the space of three days we exchanged our city life for the life of farmers in charge of a hundred and fifty animals: cows, goats, and sheep. What we actually knew about what we were doing could have balanced comfortably on a pinhead. Yet it was this very absence of knowledge that made space for real learning. When a problem arose with an animal, all we could do was look it in the eye and try to create a dialogue. To do this we had to explore subtle ways of communicating beyond the realms of language.

Gradually we felt inwardly more calm and more available, which made more space for listening to the animals. Eventually our whole system for running the farm was based on this close relationship we created with them. Looking back on this period after a space of more than twelve years, I realize it was a watershed. The change of attitude we had been compelled to make had opened up new perspectives for me, and from then on I knew I could turn the ideas which interested me in other areas into real experience. Thus I turned my attention again to trees, with the intention of trying out the approach we had learned from our dealings with the animals.

After leaving the farm we went to live in a simple hut in the depths of the forest in central France, about a thousand metres (three thousand feet) up in a range of mountains. When we went out we were surrounded by huge tracts of forest, without any roads or buildings or walkers. The trees were there waiting, it seemed, just for us, ready to share their secrets. They held out their arms to us expectantly; all we had to do was to go forward and meet them.

But how do you meet a tree? It stands in front of you, unmoving, in all its simplicity and power, and it seems to expect nothing, to be almost indifferent. All the usual props for communication vanish. At first we could only look at the trees and and observe without getting much further. We then began to make use of our other senses; we touched the trees, we smelled them, we tasted the buds and the sap when it was feasible. We put an ear to the trunk to confirm that all was quiet as we expected, and to our amazement we heard sounds and noises. Everything we tried gave us great surprises. What we expected to be bitter turned out to be syrupy, what we thought would be sweet was in fact sour, what we assumed to be stiff was actually flexible. To discover the truth of the tree we had to be open to experience what was actually there in front of us. Only through this narrow gate could we gain access to the pathway of discovery and understanding.

We also had to learn to distrust our own expectations. It is so tempting when you've had an interesting experience to try to repeat it, but this doesn't leave any space for new discoveries. In our next phase of experimenting we sat with our backs against the trees, sometimes settling ourselves as comfortably as in an armchair against their rough bark and spreading roots. With our backs to the trunk we discovered that our physical sensations changed and shifted, and by going from one tree and one kind to another we were able to map out the shifts in our physical condition and energy state

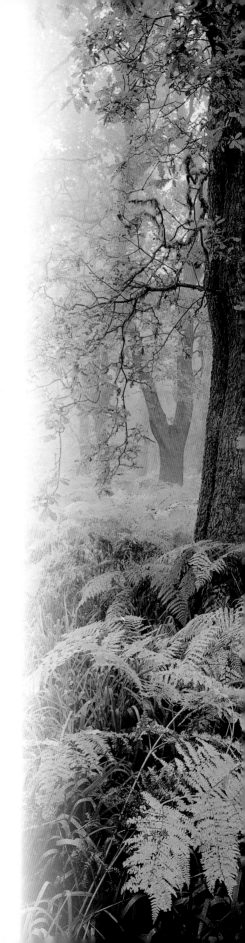

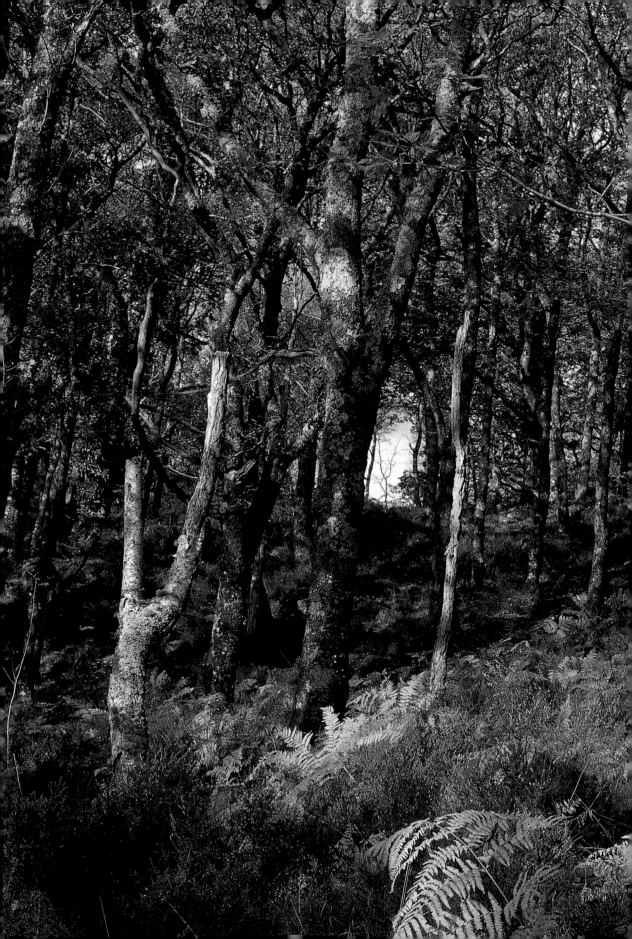

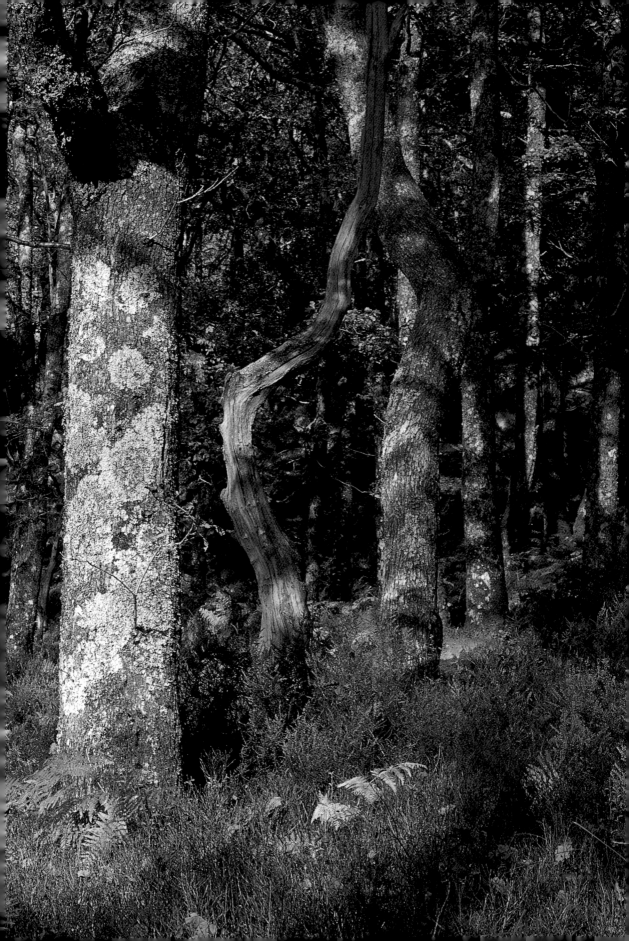

triggered by this contact, which we felt quite specifically in our own bodies. How often our breathing rhythm changed after a few minutes' leaning back against a tree, how often aches and pains vanished, how often the digestive passages moved more freely.

We also noticed the effect of the trees on our inner state. We would come with a heavy heart to a wild cherry and go away with it lightened, we would come exhausted to a pine tree and go away full of energy again, we would come to a beech tree in a turmoil of doubt, and leave it with a quiet mind. These effects were more than transitory, lasting much longer than we expected, and after a while we learned to work with them systematically.

Then we had to assimilate all the surprises that our experimentation had brought to us. The whole effect did not come from the tree; the contact we had with them brought together our own fields of energy and theirs, and the effects we perceived arose from this meeting.

We came to realize that each tree contains a certain kind of energy and that this energy varies from one species to another; some trees have an effect that encourages fluidity, with others it might be gentleness or openness. For more than ten years now we have been preparing tree oils that embody these qualities of energy. They are a wonderful support for people who want to find a new way to take care of themselves, and who are willing to learn from their problems and gain from them the true benefits of experience.

This book is an invitation for you to share the healing energies of trees. It does not present facts about trees, but offers you techniques and exercises that you can use to initiate experiences of your own. Experience is the best teacher, the door through which we gradually discover the truth about ourselves and our world. How you use the exercises will determine what fruits you harvest from your experiences.

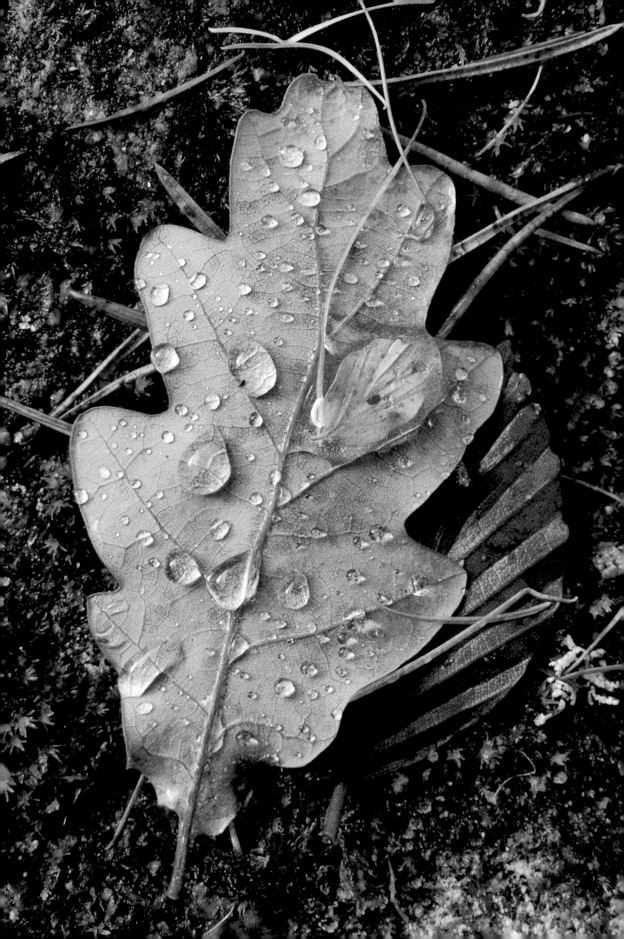

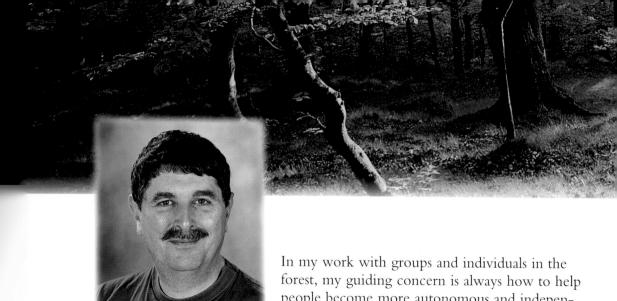

Personal note

In my work with groups and individuals in the forest, my guiding concern is always how to help people become more autonomous and independent, so they can break through their conditioning and make contact with the consciousness to which humans and nature owe their life.

The exercises in this book guide you on this journey of personal development. However, even when you follow the instructions for an exercise precisely, your experience may be quite different from what you expect. Instead of asking why it did not happen as you anticipated, concentrate on what part of you has been touched by the experience and what you have felt, realized, or understood. The guiding rule is always to focus on what you actually experience; the only useful question is, "How was it for you?"

Approach each exercise with an open mind. The more you expect, the less available you are for what actually takes place, so it is best to start with an acceptance that nothing may happen. Also, do not allow regrets to distract you: "I haven't found the right tree" or "The climate here is no good for this sort of thing". Keep your mind in the present by following your curiosity about what is going on inside you and around you. The present is the only place where something new can happen.

My observations of trees are made intuitively at the energetic level, and concern qualities rather than precise botanical detail. I have made a point of talking about "trees" and not only particular species, so the exercises apply wherever in the world you live. They can be done wherever there are trees: in a wood, a copse, or a garden. Thus

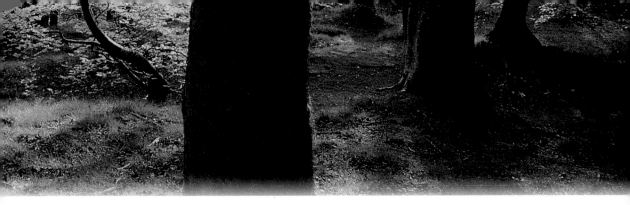

everyone can find new riches and discover more about themselves through the experience of our close connection with nature.

Chapter 1 explores our relationship with nature and how this has changed and developed since ancient times. Chapter 2 then relates our attitude to nature to our attitude to illness, as a reflection of our consciousness. The energetic structure of the body is explained, so that with an understanding of illness and healing as energetic processes we can see how the energies of trees can help us in our own healing. The exercises in Chapter 3 focus on increasing your perception of trees and discovering their healing qualities for yourself. In Chapter 4 profiles of the nine trees that I use to make my energized healing oils highlight the qualities embodied in them. Chapter 5 presents exercises and practical techniques for working with the tree energies you need to promote healing and wellbeing of body, mind, and spirit.

Take a walk into the heart of the woods. Let yourself attune to the atmosphere and the abundant life there, and you will find a source of peace and of serenity. This marvellous adventure will lead you into the heart of yourself, and in this simple intimacy you can come to understand yourself more deeply and find your true strength. Entering the domain of the trees is a wonderful way to reconnect with the life force within and around us.

Patrice Bouchardon

15

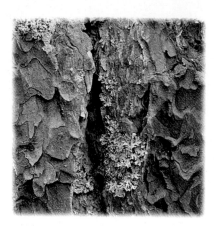

Chapter 1

What nature means to us

The two images that are most often used to symbolize nature are the tree and the flower. The flower represents nature tamed and sharing the life of man: you can plant it, cut it, bring it into the house, and invite it to be present at special occasions, whether happy or sad. Its beauty fascinates but is short-lived. The tree however is seen to represent the forest, where nature is not yet tamed or touched by the depredations of human beings.

Trees are a vital part of the inheritance of mankind. In the diversity of portrayals of the natural world in literature and philosophy, we see how great thinkers and philosphers have been both the initiators and the witnesses of the slow process of evolution which has led man from experiencing nature as something magical to be feared, to regarding it as something mechanical to be dominated. Since ancient times the tree has been a symbol of power, of wisdom, of fertility, and of life itself. Perhaps the universality of these symbols reflects something innate that connects us with the tree at a deeper level than we have imagined until now.

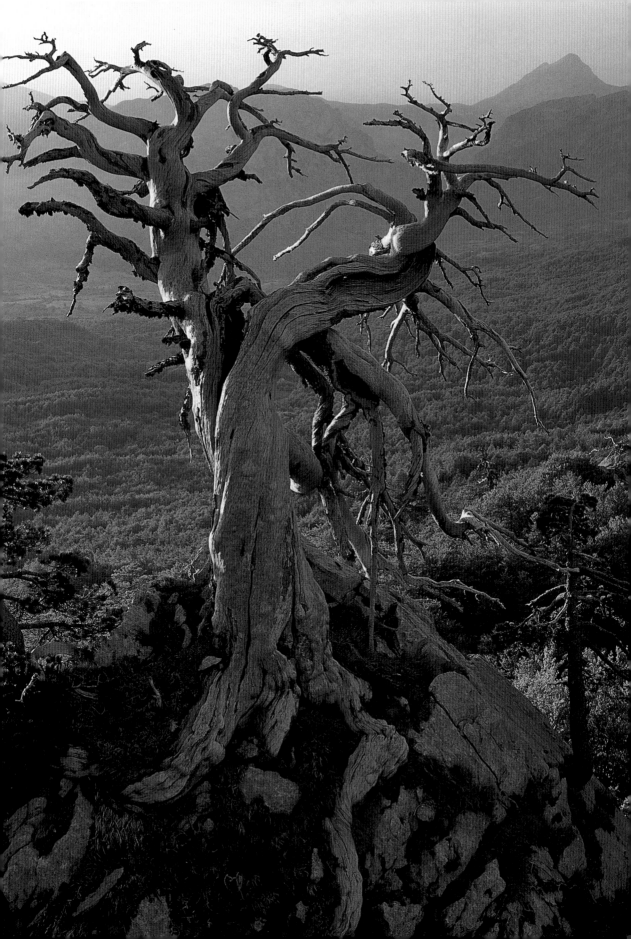

The Bible story of the Creation in the Book of Genesis tells how God planted a garden in Eden, with beautiful trees laden with delicious fruits, and placed man in it. Among them is the tree of life, symbol of immortality, and the tree of knowledge of good and evil. These two archetypal views of the tree are found in the myth, tradition, and spiritual teachings of cultures all around the world.

The tree of life

Many Creation myths focus on the tree as the powerful central element. In Norse mythology the great tree Yggdrasil was the axis of the world, its roots holding the lower world of the earth spirits together, its trunk maintaining the middle world of man, and its branches home to the upper world of the gods. In several African myths man is said to be born from a tree, and from different species in different regions. The name of the great hero of the nomadic Hottentot tribe of southwest Africa, Heitsi-Eibib, comes from the word *heigib* which means "the great tree".

In the esoteric Jewish tradition of the Kabbala, the key symbols are the sephiroth, which embody the attributes of the divine. They are represented as fruits clustered in order on the tree of life, and the links between them symbolize the stages of the soul's journey toward eternity. The Bodhi Tree under which Buddha was sitting when he attained illumination is both a classic representation of the axis of the world and a tree of life, and in the early iconography represents the Buddha himself.

For the Ismailian Shi'ite Muslims, the tree that reaches beyond the seventh heaven is the symbol of *hakikat*, the state of beatitude in which the mystic is reunited with the supreme reality. In Indian tradition God, the source of all life, is the root of the tree, while the trunk and the branches symbolize the earliest communities which grew up with a pure spirituality close to the creator. The leaves represent human beings.

With the passage of time the trunk of the tree has grown bigger and the direct link with the source has been blurred. To help mankind find the path again many prophets have come - Abraham, Buddha, Christ, Mohammed - bringing messages of peace, love, and freedom, and each one creating new branches. These branches have then further divided into smaller branches, creating a multitude of different languages, sects, cultures, religions, and "isms". Chaos reigns, suffocating the tree. However, the tree sheds seeds which carry within them the divine essence, and any one of which may become a new expression of the divine spirit.

The symbol of the tree of life contains within it a paradox: the tree draws its strength from the earth through its roots, while humans draw their strength from the divine in the heavens. This paradox is acknowledged in the many "upside down" representations of the tree of life. In the Vedic texts and the Upanishads the universe is represented as a tree upside down, spreading its roots into the sky and plunging its branches down below the earth. In these reversed images the branches act as roots and the roots as branches, bringing down the life force into the earth.

In a similar tradition the Lapplanders sacrifice a prize animal every year to the god of vegetation, and place beside the altar a tree with its roots in the air and its crown on the ground. Likewise the medicine men of certain Australian tribes used in their ceremonies a magic tree which they planted upside down as a symbolic gesture.

The foliage that falls and reappears with each yearly cycle typifies eternal renewal and the con-tinuing evolution of life, as well as reminding us of the place of death in the life process. Many cultures have the tradition of planting a tree when a child is born. As the tree grows toward the sky it acts as a reminder of the qualities of uprightness, maturity, and responsibility.

> Thus do the generations of the earth
> Go to the grave, and issue from the womb,
> Surviving still the imperishable change
> That renovates the world; even as the leaves
> Which the keen frost-wind of the waning year
> Has scatter'd on the forest soil ...
> Till from the breathing lawn a forest springs ...

Percy Bysshe Shelley
Queen Mab, V

19

This cycle of unfailing renewal is also taken as a symbol of fertility. In parts of the Middle East, from the Mediterranean across to India, travellers sometimes come across a solitary tree by a spring, hung all over with a blossom of red handkerchiefs put there by women who are barren in the hope of altering their fate. Among the Dravidians in the south of India it is the custom to "marry" two trees as a mirror of a marriage. The couple plant two sacred trees side by side, one male and one female. Then they make an enclosure around the tree partners, so that they may flourish safely and by their fruitfulness assure the fertility of the human couple.

In the Sioux tribe of North America, and among the Bushmen and Hottentots of southwest Africa, a couple who are going to be married are first betrothed to a tree. Usually, a tree that bears fruit is chosen for the ceremony, so that the couple may share in its fertility. The Waramunga tribe of northern Australia believe that certain trees harbour the spirit of a child, tiny as a grain of sand, which may then leave its tree to enter through the navel into a woman's womb. In the Mardi Gras celebrations at Hildesheim in Germany, women were traditionally hit with fir branches so that they would bear children.

"If the tree be good then its fruit shall be good; if the tree be bad then its fruit shall be bad likewise. For by its fruit is the tree known."

The Bible
Matthew XII, v. 33

The tree of knowledge

Trees are often associated with the gift of wisdom. Saint Louis, king of France in the 13th century and renowned for his virtue and integrity, meted out justice sitting beneath an oak tree. In many African communities a special tree is designated as the "talking tree", and it is here that the elders gather to hold their lengthy discussions of village affairs.

Wisdom arises from the knowledge of good and evil, and from this concept the tree has also emerged as a symbol of peace. In the days when the Iroquois nation in North America lived in anarchy and division, a man called Peacemaker

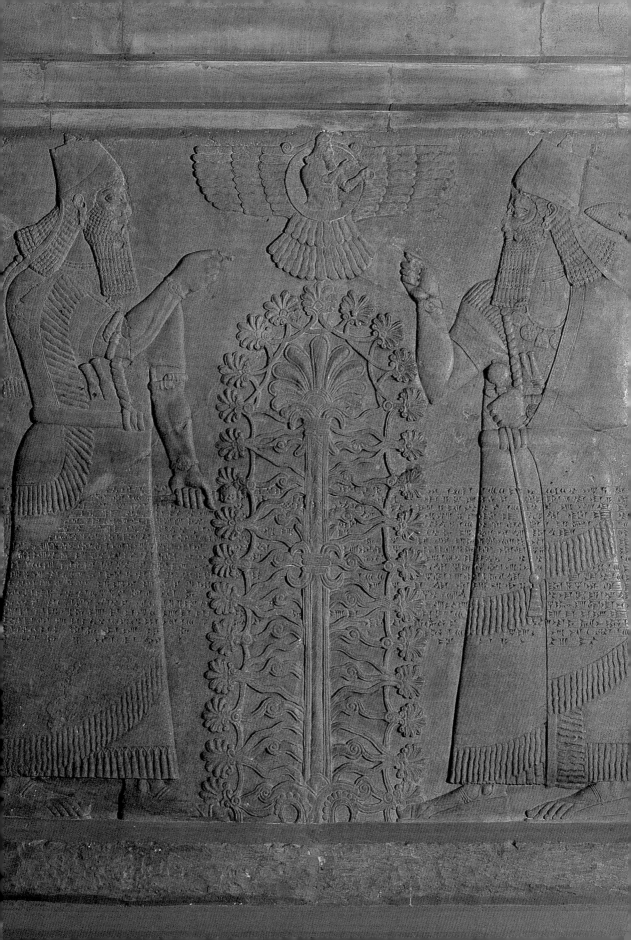

The tree within us

In the human body many distribution systems are organized around a structure reminiscent of a tree. The blood circulates from the heart, the root, and from there branches into the arteries, veins, and smaller blood vessels in ever finer ramifications. Likewise in the respiratory system air enters the body through the nasal passages and travels through the bronchi, which branch into the multiple alveoli of the lungs. The messages of the nervous system too are radiated out from the brain and the spinal cord through the major nerves and then through ever smaller nerve bundles, to reach every part of the body. And then there is the return traffic; the flow returns toward the point of origin as the life force returns from the finest roots and the furthest twigs back toward the trunk.

❷ *In a given situation which prompts an emotional response we tend to react in the same way. This habit of reaction becomes the trunk of our behaviour pattern.*

❶ *The same model of the tree can be used to illustrate our mental and emotional processes. An emotion is always triggered by an event or experience which seems to be the reason why we feel as we do, while in fact the true reason, the root cause of our sensitivity, is out of sight in the unconscious, as the tree roots are hidden in the earth.*

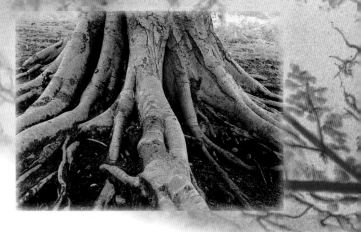

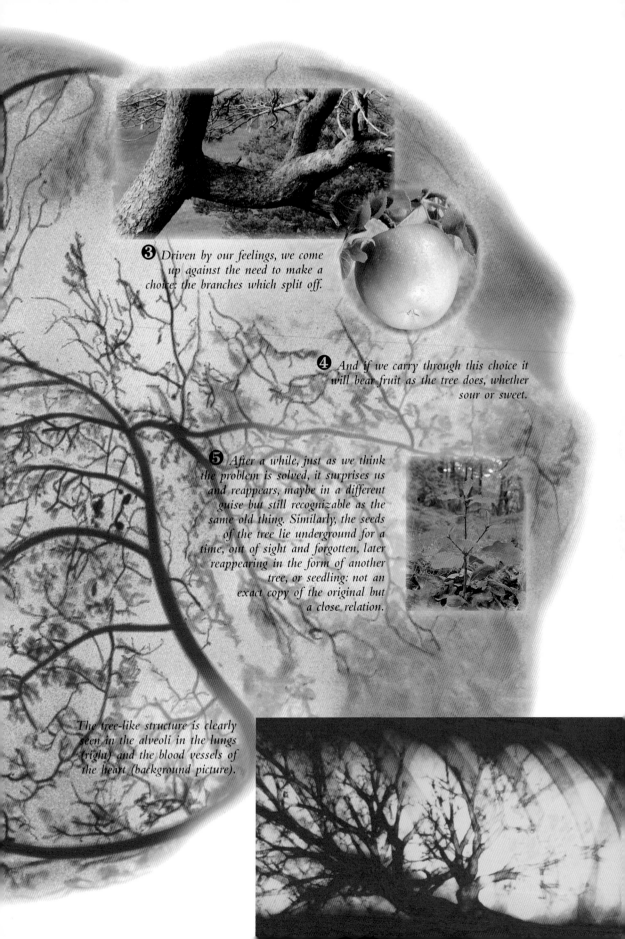

❸ *Driven by our feelings, we come up against the need to make a choice: the branches which split off.*

❹ *And if we carry through this choice it will bear fruit as the tree does, whether sour or sweet.*

❺ *After a while, just as we think the problem is solved, it surprises us and reappears, maybe in a different guise but still recognizable as the same old thing. Similarly, the seeds of the tree lie underground for a time, out of sight and forgotten, later reappearing in the form of another tree, or seedling: not an exact copy of the original but a close relation.*

The tree-like structure is clearly seen in the alveoli in the lungs (right) and the blood vessels of the heart (background picture).

came to them. He brought all the leaders of the warring factions together by the shores of Lake Onondaga for the first council of reconciliation, where after much talking the five different nations agreed to be united into one.

As a symbol of this new nation Peacemaker chose the white pine, since its tufts of needles, five in each one, represented the five nations now united. He dug up a white pine growing nearby, revealing a great hole, in whose depths ran a river. All the assembled leaders threw their weapons into this river, and then Peacemaker closed the hole and replanted above it the white pine, which had four mighty roots spreading out to each of the four directions. He told them that anyone who wished for peace could follow one of these directions and so find refuge beneath the great tree of peace.

This peace lasted for several centuries, until the arrival of the European colonizers. In June 1776, ambassadors from the Iroquois contributed their ideas on liberty, the law, democracy and government to a nationwide congress in Philadelphia. Three weeks later the Declaration of Independence was signed and the new democracy was born. The white pine became the symbol of the newly united states, a unique emblem of government, symbolizing federation and a reminder that peace is part of the natural order.

Trees are often planted at the birth of a new era. In France, after the Revolution between 1789 and 1792, sixty thousand Trees of Liberty were planted. Belgians planted trees to celebrate their independence in 1830. And various countries have adopted trees as their national emblem. Canada has a maple leaf blazoned on the national flag; Lebanon is known by its noble cedar. The state of Illinois voted in 1907 to adopt the white oak as its emblem, and the province of the Transvaal in South Africa chose the baobab.

The tree also features in company logos as a symbol of prosperity and expansion. Computer companies Apple and Bull use the tree as a symbol of communication, a reminder of the tree structure underlying the organization of information in a computer system. The image of the tree is also used to show a company's commitment to the natural environment.

Tree traditions

The Japanese mark the New Year week by putting two pine trees of the same height on each side of the front door. According to Shinto tradition, the divinities live among the branches of trees, so the pine trees are placed in the hope of attracting them and their blessings to the house. Since ancient times many cultures have celebrated the shortest day of the year and the triumph of light over darkness. The Egyptians decorated their houses with palm leaves at this time and the Romans brought branches of evergreens into their homes for the winter festival of Saturnalia. In the Middle Ages the approach of the Feast of the Nativity was the signal to go into the forest and cut down a pine tree to put up in the house. Thus Christianity incorporated an ancient tradition where the rebirth of light after the midwinter darkness was linked with an evergreen tree, which symbolized the continuity of life.

The first specific reference to this pine tree as a "Christmas tree" dates from the 16th century, when it was the custom in Strasbourg to decorate the trees with coloured paper, fruit, and painted eggs. Gradually this custom spread across the globe: German settlers, and the Hessian mercenaries fighting in the Civil War, imported the custom to the US, where in 1804 soldiers at Fort Dearborn hauled trees from the woods to their barracks at Christmas time. The German princess Helen von Mecklenburg, wife of King Louis Philippe's son, introduced the tradition to the French court in 1840, while Prince Albert, the German husband of Queen Victoria, brought the idea to England.

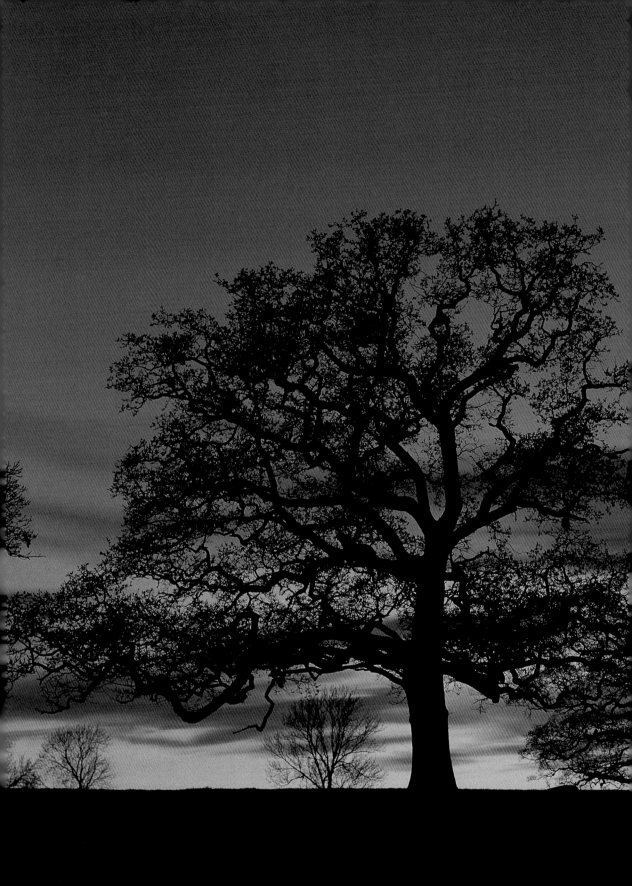

Visions of nature

Nature, or rather the idea of nature that we create for ourselves, is not the same for each of us. Throughout history man has moved forward between the pulls of two opposing attitudes: the spiritual and the materialist. The persistent ambition to dominate nature is one interpretation of the mythic images of Apollo slaying the serpent Python, and St George defeating the dragon. Man has exercised his power in the materialist struggle against the forces of nature.

The spiritual view focuses on the living and spiritual aspects of nature, and the belief that the gods, or higher powers, created the natural world and sustain all that lives within it. Natural phenomena are seen as the acting out of the will and the power of these gods. A good harvest is a reward while storm, wind, and hail are witness of their anger. All of the indigenous peoples of the world have built up cultures and social structures framed around their concepts of nature, concepts woven from their direct experience of the natural world. They draw from the world about them those things they need to sustain life, to feed and to heal the body, and to build the beliefs that nourish the soul. From this inexhaustible resource come their concepts of life and inspiration for healing and religious practices.

This magical nature, as something to be feared, is seen in the ancient European myths peopled by gods and goddesses, which reflect man's efforts to find an order and structure in nature. Socrates, and later Aristotle, rejected this "magical" view, preferring to concentrate on the order they perceived in the natural world, based on principles of beauty and logic and governed by the idea of the good.

By the Middle Ages a view prevalent among philosophers and theologians was that nature was created by God for man, but independent of him.

May my hands respect the things you have made, may my ears be attentive to your voice.

Make me wise so I can know those things you have taught my people, the lessons you have hidden in each leaf and each stone.

Amerindian prayer

And here begins the split that separates man from the rest of the natural world. In the writings of the ancient Greeks, Renaissance thinkers discovered theories that rivalled the accepted Bible version of the Creation. Nature was no longer to be regarded in reverent awe. Its multitudinous diversity was open to investigation, experiment, and explanation, in the terms of the new sciences of chemistry, physics, anatomy, mathematics, and astronomy.

The Renaissance was a period of re-evaluation of the place of man in relation to nature and to God, and fundamentally altered the European world-view. The materialist view came to the fore: of the natural world as an assortment of separate phenomena, and the work of the scientist being to discover some kind of coherence that could link them together. But in this scientific investigation certain fundamental needs of the human psyche are ignored: the ancient need to perceive the magical power of nature and feel one has a place within it, needs which came to the surface centuries later in the Romantic movement (see right).

In the 19th century, armed with the new technologies, the developing industrial nations' drive to dominate nature took on the ruthlessness of conquest. All too often it was in a bloodbath that "civilized" man took away land from native peoples: the Amerindians in northern and southern America, the Aborigines in Australia, and the Maoris in New Zealand. By destroying peoples who live in harmony with the spiritual aspects of nature, man the predator also destroys his own spiritual dimension. This destruction of the living link with nature is now a part of the collective history and consciousness of mankind.

An increasing number of scientists, working from the insights of the physicist Fritjof Capra, are realizing that the ancient spiritual concepts provide a coherent framework for the most recent scientific theories. Nature is an indivisible whole, made up of relationships that are part of a cosmic process.

THE ROMANTIC MOVEMENT

The Romantic view of nature focuses on aesthetics. It does not differentiate matter and spirit, but welcomes the emotion awakened by the experience of the natural world - an experience that prompts neither analysis nor prayer, but feeling. This aesthetic response inspires the work of all artists who marvel at the glories of a sunset or the majesty of a tree.

The Romantic movement in the 18th and 19th centuries was a reaction to the material-ist attitudes prevalent at the time. The issue was no longer whether spirit or matter ruled in nature, but to respond to the powerful emotions it evokes. Such emotion can be seen in the works of the French writers Diderot and Rousseau, in the paintings of Boucher and Fragonard, the visionary landscapes of Samuel Palmer, and in the passionate lives and works of Blake, Shelley, Keats, Wordsworth, and Byron.

The effects of destruction

By ignoring the soul of nature, the materialist attitude opened the way for humans to dominate and exploit the vast storehouse of natural resources. In the 19th century clearing forests was regarded as a local issue between colonizers and the people they invaded. But it can also be seen as a manifestation of the conflict between the material and spiritual view of nature.

This conflict is still much in evidence today. Powerful commercial interests are threatening all the world's forests. Every year we cut down or burn 17 million hectares (42 million acres) of forest – an area four times the size of Switzerland. The burning of the Amazon forest is on such a scale that the smoke from it can be seen from miles above the Earth. This burning produces carbon dioxide, contributing to the greenhouse effect which is causing climatic change and making the planet hotter.

Deforestation is an enormous danger for the ecosystems of the whole planet. Plant and animal species are destroyed along with their habitat, agricultural land is eroded, and both the local and regional climate may be affected, leading to extremes of drought or flooding. The forests are the planet's lungs, absorbing carbon dioxide and giving out oxygen. Thus local destruction has a global effect: the poisoning and destruction of the forests is something that involves us all.

Trees provide tomorrow's protection

Motto of the Nebraska tree conservation programme

Reconciliation

Nowadays, some aspects of the materialist approach and this separation from nature concern us deeply because they affect the way we live. The food industry produces food which has lost its natural flavours, we are becoming aware that medicines we take to heal us may have harmful side effects, and the spread of vast cities cuts us off from the land. In the face of all this we are now witnessing a tremendous demand for something that is genuine, authentic, and natural. There is an ever deeper

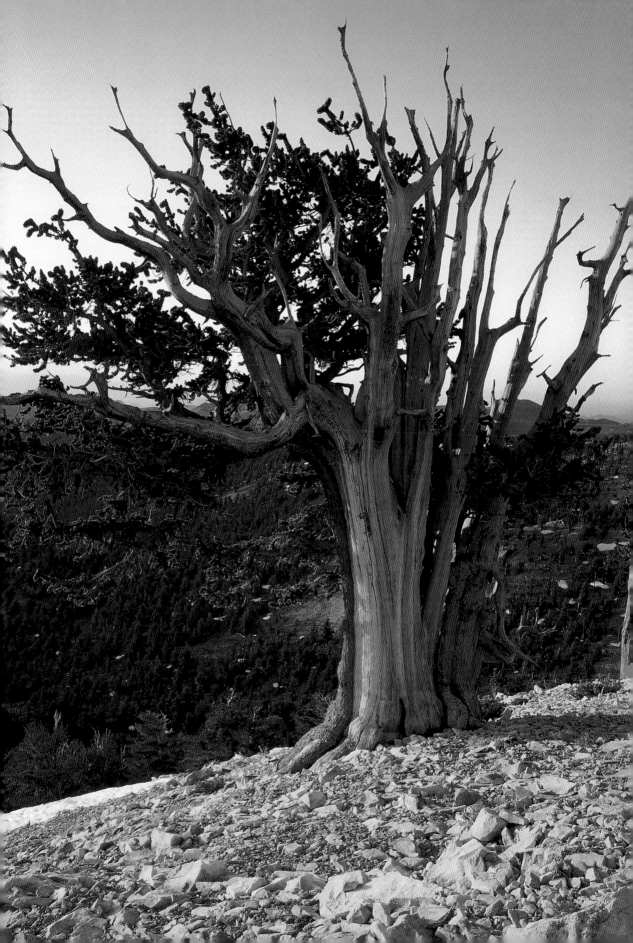

awareness of how essential it is for our wellbeing and our balance to return to a closeness with the natural world.

Now that new technologies are giving the wealthy in the industrialized system more choice about how and where they work, the aim of many city dwellers is to leave town to live in more rural areas. There is a growing interest in medical practices which have not lost sight of humans' place in nature, such as the Chinese, Tibetan, or Ayurvedic traditions. Consumer demand has led to a greater choice of organic produce being available on the supermarket shelves. Leisure activities are focused on spending more time in the open and in more remote places on the globe, whether it's rafting down tropical torrents, birdwatching in northern summers, or trekking across distant deserts.

This desire to return to our place in the natural environment is having an impact on policy making too. The influence of environmental campaigners and pressure groups, and "green" political parties, is compelling all politicians to take measures to ensure that development respects the natural world and its traditional guardians.

The New Zealand government is returning their lands to the Maoris and levying a special tax on the properties built on land that is traditionally theirs but cannot be returned. The revenues so raised are going towards establishing cultural centres and schools in order to help the Maori people reconnect with their roots. In Australia the government has set up the Council for Aboriginal Reconciliation with the aim of creating "a united Australia which respects this land of ours; values the Aboriginal and Torres Strait Islander heritage; and provides justice and equity for all" and which affirms "the unique position of indigenous Australians as the original inhabitants of this continent". There are similar developments in Canada, with the offical recognition of the Inuit people and the creation of a Foundation for Respect.

Getting back in touch with nature

Most of us are so used to seeing trees somewhere in our surroundings that we take them for granted, until they begin to decay or get sick. No-one who sees the terrible decay of the trees in the Black Forest in Germany can help wondering how much more damage pollution is going to cause now and in the future. These gaunt skeletons bear the marks of our attitude to the life of the planet; their sickness shows all too clearly the state of our relationship to the natural world. But apart from the dire warnings conveyed by the trees that are suffering, those we see around us in good health and in beauty offer us a continuing reminder of the richness of the living world. Woods and forests still provide a special place for finding peace, silence, beauty; precious qualities that are becoming more and more needed to combat the stress of daily life.

Our western "supermarket" lifestyle can sometimes make us forget that the natural world is the fundamental source of our life on Earth. It provides our food, our clothes, our medicines, the raw materials for our houses, for our heating, for synthetic pharmaceuticals, and for the thousand and one things we need in everyday life. But it still has secrets that we have not yet discovered.

The natural world offers us another precious gift: a place to live in that suits our physical and psychological make-up. How could we survive if there were extreme changes of temperature, if the Sun stopped shining or shone all the time, if all the trees disappeared? Deforestation is the tragic symbol of the ecological damage that threatens our future. It doesn't only affect the forest dweller in Brazil, but each of us, wherever we live. As you come to value contact with trees, what is happening to the world's forests becomes not just data from afar but something you care about deeply. Trees with their majestic presence remind us that the mysteries of life are beyond our grasp and to understand them better we must first respect life.

> We do not inherit the world from our parents, we borrow it from our children.
>
> *Traditional Amerindian saying*

Attitudes to nature

Each of us has a personal relationship with nature and with trees. The seven most common attitudes are described below.

In Chapter 2 you will discover how your attitudes to illness and to nature reflect your attitude to life as a whole, and the stage you are at in your own personal development.

❶ THE "FARMER"

The farmer views nature - animals, trees, land - as a source of production or profit to be exploited. Plants and animals are something apart from himself, requiring no more contact than is necessary to keep them in order and dominate them.
"Real trees are a renewable, recyclable resource. Artificial treees contain non-biodegradable plastics and metals."
The American National Christmas Tree Association
The real tree is presented as an "ecological object" but essentially as a raw material.

❷ THE "BIOLOGIST"

The biologist does not feel any direct link with the tree but is curious to understand "how it works": where it grows, how it reproduces; the facts, the identifying details. The tree and the living being are mechanisms which can be dismantled into constituent parts. It is the classic mechanistic view of nature.
"... a vast decrease in the world population ... is the only way to eliminate poverty and stop such ecological disasters as the greenhouse effect and the destruction of the rainforest and with them the habitat for ever-dwindling plants and animals."
May Drake, Teacher, UK
Visions of a better world

❸ THE "ROMANTIC"

The romantic sees how man makes nature suffer, and suffers with it. For him, nature is the domain where all is beautiful, all is pure, and it is man who is the destroyer. He finds in nature a longed-for refuge.
"So I went slowly on, looking for some wild place in the forest, a place untouched where there was no sign of the slavery of domination that man creates, some sheltered spot which I could believe I was the first to set foot in."
Jean-Jacques Rousseau

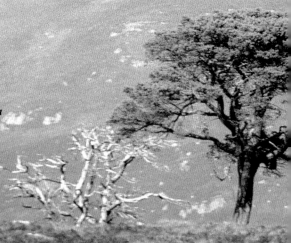

❹ THE "GARDENER"

The gardener has a friendly, uncomplicated relationship with plants and trees. When she is with them she feels she is among old friends. She marvels at the beauty of nature, but without projecting her own feeling onto what she sees. Her love is not overloaded with emotion. The person with this attitude is often actually a gardener, known for her "green fingers".

"I would like nature to be a green nature, with green grasses, with lots of flower gardens and trees in which the birds fly. I would like a nature with a light wind in the trees to bring a fresh breeze."
Godelieve Uwinama, Student, Rwanda
Visions of a better world

❺ THE "SHAMAN"

The shaman goes out into nature to restore her energy, without understanding how this works. However, she feels deep down, without being able to say why, that the forest is a living theatre. Often she has experiences that overwhelm her, she talks to the trees and hears answers, she sees things that others do not. She often hugs a tree, which soothes her soul.

"Each path and track has its own sensitivity and psychic existence, shaped by the consciousness of those who have made it and used it. That's why some old roads have a strong energetic personality and can give rise to certain states of being, making one open to the inspiration of the spirit of the place."
Nathalie and Michel Vogt,
La forêt du Rhin
secrète et légendaire

❻ THE "ECOLOGIST"

It is through his inner awareness that the ecologist understands the tree and the natural world. His knowledge is not the result of a mental or intellectual process, but of a deep inner experience. He is conscious that the tree is more than it seems to be, and he glimpses within himself its other dimensions. For him nature is an unending source of beauty and of ecstasy.

"My vision of the world is one in which man has reached the point of understanding that he is not the owner of nature but forms a part of her. The balance between man and nature is essential to the possibility of life on this planet."
Emanuel, Singer, Mexico
Visions of a better world

❼ THE "MYSTIC"

The mystic perceives what he and the tree have in common. For him the tree is a transcendent creation, and the contact with it enables him to connect with the divine in himself. He knows that the destiny of man and of nature are not only linked, but are the expression of one and the same thing.

*"My words are tied in one
With the great mountains,
With the great rocks,
With the great trees,
In one with my body
And my heart"*
Yokuts Indian Prayer

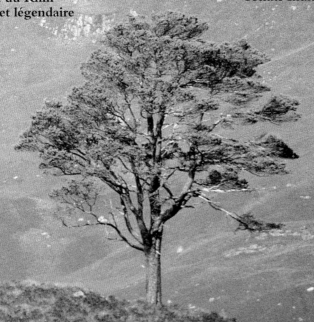

To understand the usefulness of this typology it must be understood that the categories are not rigid. Your viewpoint varies according to what you are facing at any time. For example, in the same situation you can react as a farmer one time and at another time as a romantic. Within each category there are highs and lows. Thus the "farmer", who sees the tree primarily as a resource to be used, may use it in different ways: for his own profit, to make a beautiful object or something that other people need, or to share generously with others. In fact at each level there are two polarities, which indicate the extremes of attitude on each level. If we want to improve and develop ourselves and rise to a higher level of awareness, we will find our-selves impelled to move through each level from the starting-point of one polarity to the attainment of the other.

The progression from one polarity to its opposite usually happens slowly, while a shift up to another level often means a sudden break with the old pattern of behaviour. For example, a move from farmer to biologist involves a change of focus. The idea of using up nature's resources without a second thought suddenly becomes repellent.

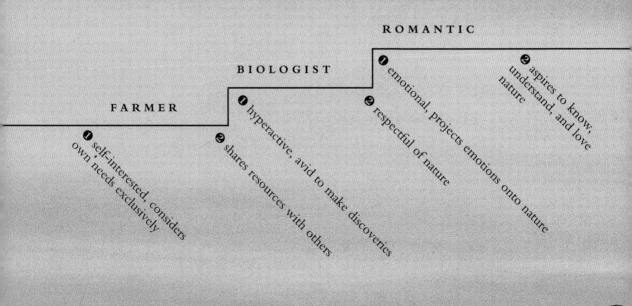

ROMANTIC

BIOLOGIST

FARMER

❶ self-interested, considers own needs exclusively

❷ shares resources with others

❶ hyperactive, avid to make discoveries

❷ respectful of nature

❶ emotional, projects emotions onto nature

❷ aspires to know, understand, and love nature

TYPE OF ATTITUDE TO NATURE	ATTITUDE TO TREES
FARMER	a resource to be exploited
BIOLOGIST	objects to investigate
ROMANTIC	beings that mirror our own suffering
GARDENER	beings to take care of
SHAMAN	a source of power
ECOLOGIST	living beings
MYSTIC	part of the cosmic whole

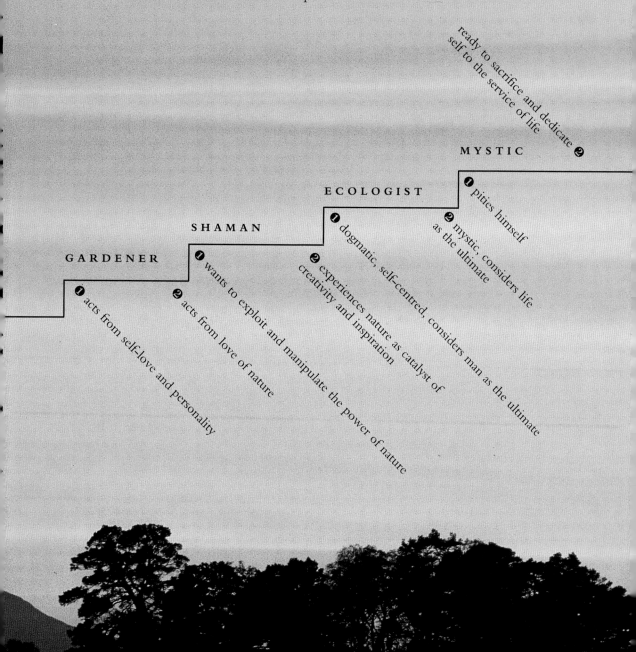

MYSTIC

ECOLOGIST

SHAMAN

GARDENER

ready to sacrifice and dedicate self to the service of life

pities himself

mystic, considers life as the ultimate

dogmatic, self-centred, considers man as the ultimate

experiences nature as catalyst of creativity and inspiration

wants to exploit and manipulate the power of nature

acts from love of nature

acts from self-love and personality

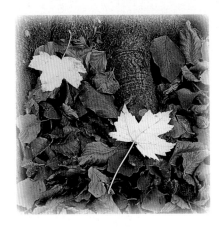

Chapter 2

The healing process

The first step in understanding how trees can help you is to look at yourself and your problems from a new perspective. To some people it's a new idea, to others an ancient truth, that a human being is not just a physical body to which a spirit has been added. Rather a human is essentially a spirit, an energetic presence, or energy body, dwelling in a physical frame. The exercises in this chapter will help you become more aware of this energy body, its structure, and how it interacts with the physical body.

We have a good understanding of the process of illness in the physical body, but we need to become more aware of the processes in the energy body. In fact physical symptoms, and mental or emotional problems, are often facets of the same inner state. By looking at physical, mental, and emotional crises in terms of their energetic effects it is possible to identify a sequence of stages of the healing process. With this understanding you will realize that you are not the helpless victim in your illness or problem, but that you have in your grasp the key to your healing and growth.

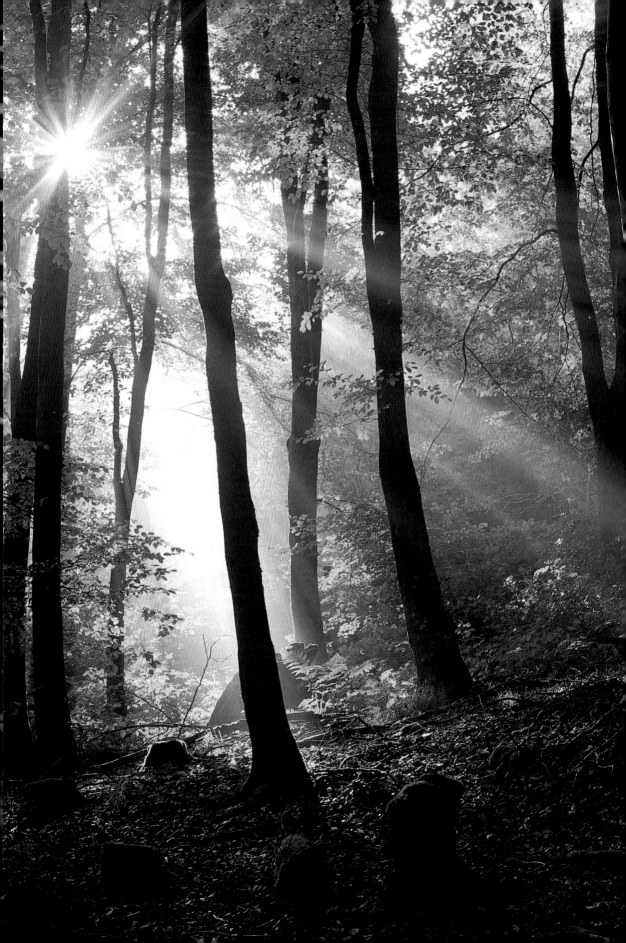

Attitudes to illness

From my experiences with working with people and in my workshops I have observed seven common attitudes to illness that parallel the attitudes to nature described in Chapter 1.

Most people have a mixture of these attitudes, and will go through a range of reactions in a given situation, though probably one pattern will predominate. For example, someone might show "ecologist" tendencies at one moment and those of the "farmer" at another. The attitude will only apply to that problem at that one precise moment.

❶ THE FARMER

This person notices the illness only when it becomes a hindrance or the pain is really bad. Its parallel is the "farmer" attitude to nature, only taking notice of nature in its most obvious aspects and seeing it as a resource to be used. The abundance of the natural world just appears in front of him as a source of something useful, and an illness appears likewise, but as a source of trouble.

❷ THE BIOLOGIST

This person reacts by trying to explain what is happening as the result of an outside cause. "What virus is doing this to me?" "Have I eaten some bad food?" "I've inherited this tendency to depression from my mother." Similarly, in their attitude to nature biologists try to understand and find the reasons for things but assume they are "out there".

❸ THE ROMANTIC

Romantics feel their illness is a personal insult, the sure indication of their bad luck or that fate is unfair, and they react with strong feelings. The parallel attitude to nature is to see in it a passionate suffering that they want to be involved in.

❹ THE GARDENER

The gardener has a practical attitude and relates to nature through active involvement. In the same way they deal with illness practically: when indications of disease appear they give up smoking, change their diet, take up sport, or whatever else makes them feel more in tune with the body.

❺ THE SHAMAN

People with this attitude imagine that to cure their illness there must be some powerful remedy or healing method available somewhere, other than that offered by their doctor. This parallels their attitude to nature, which they imagine as a storehouse of powerful forces.

❻ THE ECOLOGIST

When these people become ill they take time to consider what has brought them to this situation and what it reveals about their way of life. In a similar way "ecologists" seek to understand the natural world through their inner experiences.

❼ THE MYSTIC

Mystics feel that their own health imbalance reflects their personal share in a collective process of evolution and transformation. They view their experience in the context of the whole of humanity, just as they understand themselves to be part of nature.

EXERCISE 1: *EXPLORING YOUR ATTITUDE TO YOUR OWN ILLNESS*

This exercise will help you to focus on your attitude during illness and realize what your expectations are about getting through it.

When you get ill, what do you experience?
What do you feel?
What is your emotional or mental attitude to your illness?

How do you expect to get better?

How far do you feel responsible for your illness or for what has happened?

Can you imagine having a different attitude to your illness?
What could it be?
What difference could this attitude make in the rest of your life?

What implications does this have for your relationship with your doctor or therapist?

41

The parallels between the attitudes to nature described in Chapter 1, and the attitudes to illness, indicate a link between them. Both these attitudes are reflections that indicate the angle of our own personal mirror that we hold up to life: how we have learned to orientate our processes of perception and the conclusions we have drawn from our experience of life through these perceptions. All this is filed in our consciousness: the storehouse of our inner perceptions, our feelings, our thoughts, the harvest of our memories, the perception of our physical body, the way in which we experience the world around us, our sense of beauty, of good and evil, of our spiritual aspirations.

Although conventional science has yet to find an explanation, ancient traditions from different cultures have explained where our consciousness resides in similar terms: at different levels in our energy bodies.

The energy bodies

Why is it that when we are faced with a situation that rouses strong feelings, we suddenly have a lump in the throat that stops us from saying anything? Conversely, when we are in pain, or suffering physically, it is hard to think clearly. Strong emotions and feelings can likewise cloud the mind, and hinder or block our mental and physical faculties.

Clearly there is something that carries this information between our thoughts, our feelings, and our physical body. The connection is made through our energy bodies, in some traditions called the subtle bodies. These "bodies" are composed of energy: they are not dense like the physical body, so we cannot feel their substance, but we do feel their effects, their workings, and their exchanges of information. Since they each have the same centre as the physical body, changes within them can affect the physical body and vice versa.

THE ENERGY BODIES AND THEIR AURAS

❶ The physical body, the one we know best, which is the sole focus of interest for most scientific researchers and doctors.

❷ The emotional or astral body: the body filled by our emotions.

❸ The mental body: the body composed of our thoughts.

❹ The causal body holds the memory of our entire soul experience.

❺ The spiritual bodies: our true nature. Through these bodies we are connected with the plane of universal life.

The ego, made up of the physical, emotional, and mental bodies, holds our familiar patterns of thinking and acting.

The higher self, made up of the causal and spiritual bodies, is the source of our inner wisdom.

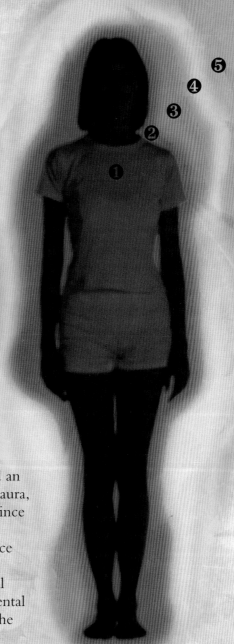

Each energy body has a field of radiance called an aura: the emotional body emits the emotional aura, the mental body the mental aura, and so on. Since each energy body has a characteristic range of vibration they are able to exist in the same space simultaneously. The higher the vibration, the greater the extent of the aura, so the emotional aura extends beyond the physical body, the mental aura radiates beyond the emotional aura, and the causal and spiritual auras radiate further still.

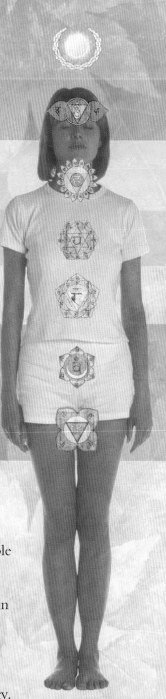

THE SEVEN MAIN CHAKRAS AND THEIR RELATED ENERGIES

❼ Crown – *spiritual connection*

❻ Ajna, third eye – *intelligence, perception*

❺ Throat – *expression, communication*

❹ Heart centre – *love*

❸ Solar plexus – *emotions*

❷ Hara – *close relationships, sexuality*

❶ Coccyx – *basic life instincts*

The seven main chakras

The energy bodies are made up of a web of invisible energy channels, known by their Sanskrit name *nadis*. Where these channels cross each other they form vortices of energy called chakras. At the main meeting-points dozens of *nadis* come together, creating seven major chakras (see illustration), through which information can flow between the energy bodies and along all the channels. Each chakra is the focal point of a certain type of energy.

Becoming aware of energy bodies

Our differences are obvious in our physical bodies, in skin colour, hair texture, features, and so on. Apart from a few identical doubles, we do not look like our neighbours. But we are more alike in our emotional bodies: the anger you feel is much the same as that felt by anyone else on the planet. Our patterns of thinking are even more alike, although the things we think about are very different.

Generally we are aware more or less of our physical bodies, less so of our feelings, less still of our thinking patterns, and not at all of our spiritual nature. When I talk about being aware, I mean recognizing the true nature of our feelings and our thoughts. We think we know about them because we live with their effects, but this does not mean we understand them fully, any more than we can claim to understand light because we know how to press a switch to light a bulb.

The exercise below will help you become aware of your energy bodies.

EXERCISE 2: *LEARNING TO DETECT THE ENERGY BODIES*

❶ Settle in a comfortable place, close your eyes, and put your palms together. Slowly move your hands apart, noticing carefully your sensations. When they are close you may feel some connection between them, but as they move further apart you will notice that this connection breaks and you feel nothing more.

❷ At this point begin to bring your hands closer again very slowly, and you will probably have a sense of something resilient between them, like a bouncy balloon.

❸ Explore these sensations and notice what you feel - heat, cold, pins and needles, a pull together, a resistance. Then separate your hands further until you feel the next break, and explore this in the same way.

45

Listening to your energy bodies

You might wonder how it helps us to know about energy bodies, when our thoughts and feelings are already familiar to us from their effects on our daily life. Generally, in solving a problem, the mind takes charge of the operation, but it is all too easy to let yourself be tricked by your mind. So many generally accepted ideas shape our belief systems without our realizing it and prevent us from free thinking: the religious belief that certain people will be saved and others will not; the belief that everything "scientific" must necessarily be true. We can base a whole way of behaving on a misconception, such as the idea that sometimes allowing ourselves time to concentrate on our own needs is selfish. Since the influence of these beliefs and misconceptions can be so powerful, we can glimpse the dangers of a therapy that works only on the mind level. To get a more complete picture, listen to what your energy bodies are telling you.

With some practice you can learn to register what is happening in your energy bodies, which puts you in touch with reality without any cheating. Your bodily sensations are a sure indicator of whether or not your behaviour is authentic. You might ask yourself "Am I clear in my relationship with so and so?" "Do I really have confidence in myself?" and from the sensations in your body you will get answers that may not be those your mind would come up with. Your energy bodies will give you clear hints about how to improve your relationship, come to terms with losing your job, or develop your self-confidence, without any interference from your mind. The exercise (left) shows you how to become aware of your bodily sensations; further techniques can be learned from audio cassettes (see page 160).

EXERCISE 3: *LEARNING TO LISTEN TO THE ENERGY BODIES*

Since the energy bodies share the same space as the physical body, you will be able to feel the sensations they give rise to by relaxing your physical body. The mind is present only as an observer in this exercise.

❶ Lie down comfortably and pay attention to the sensations in your body, such as heat, tension, discomfort, without trying to change any of them.

❷ When you have registered how you are in your body, think of something that gives you pleasure. Notice any changes, any inner movments or new sensations, and where they are strongest.

❸ Now let that thought go, relax again, and pay attention to your body's sensations.

❹ Bring to mind something you don't like. Notice again the sensations – are they in the same places? Do they have the same quality?

❺ Let that thought go, relax, and check your state again.

❻ Bring to mind something pleasant. Listen again to how your body responds.

❼ Relax and gradually bring yourself back to the present.

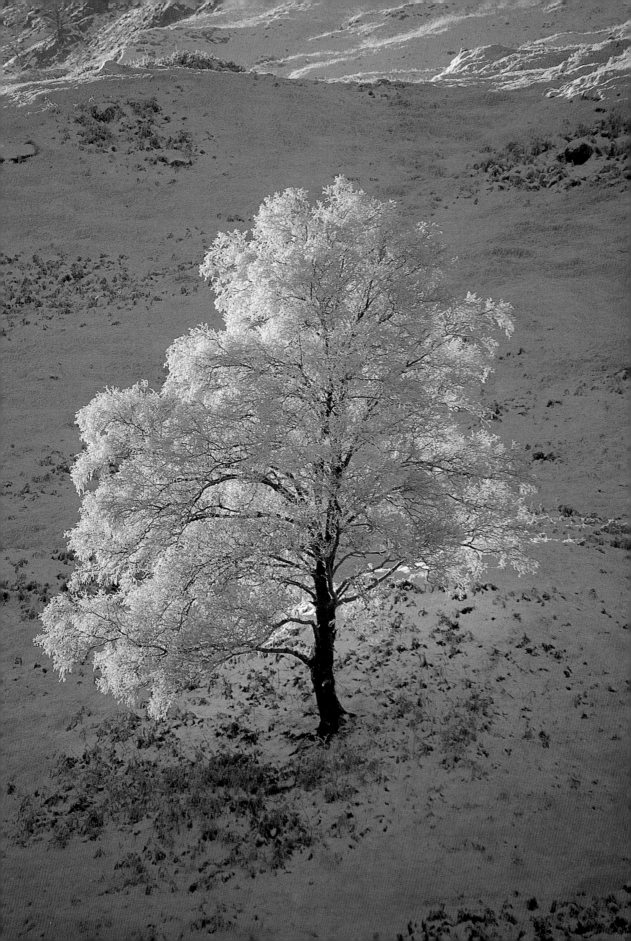

How illness arises

The vital dynamic that keeps the physical body functioning has its source in the energy bodies, so when they are weakened or out of tune the physical body cannot go on working as it should. The energy bodies are in turn governed by our inner state of being. When we are in a state of imbalance the damaging effects are caused not just by our emotions or by our thought patterns or by our physical body, but by the way they interact and feed into each other. Since the energy bodies are in continual movement and interaction with each other, a problem is not localized at a fixed point but rather is a knot or distortion in an interweaving fabric of impulses and reactions. This distortion upsets the flow of our energy bodies and creates a physical malfunction, which in turn makes us feel even worse as we go around the cycle of miserable thoughts and feelings again and again. Such a situation is illustrated in the case study (left).

All of us carry microbes and viruses and potential cancer cells in our system, but not everyone gets ill from them. A disease will only manifest when the system has a particular weakness. If the processes of the energy bodies and the physical body are out of balance, this may provide an opening for a bug or virus to invade the system.

Conventional medicine sometimes makes the mistake of focusing solely on the physical body. Energy medicine practitioners may often make the parallel mistake of trying to find the cause of the problem in the energy bodies and forgetting to check out the physical body. In fact an illness represents an interaction between the energy bodies and the physical body - or a lack of interaction - rather than a direct impact of one upon the other.

CASE STUDY

H was an attractive woman of 35, who in spite of her beauty had low self-esteem and was always looking for reassurance. She always wore flamboyant make-up and provocative clothing in an attempt to boost her confidence. For her, being a woman meant being inferior and vulnerable, so she was always battling to get the upper hand. Physically she suffered from painful and irregular periods, and involuntary contraction of the vagina, so that sexual intimacy was painful.

Her feelings and beliefs due to her sense of weakness as a woman had created in her energy bodies a whirlpool of energy in the belly area that drew in all around it, thus preventing her other energies from circulating freely. This dense blockage made her hold back unconsciously everything that might remind her that she was a woman: hence the painful periods and vaginal contractions. In turn these physical symptoms caused her more fearful and negative thoughts of herself, reinforcing the distorted energy pattern.

The functions of illness

For most of us getting over an illness means getting rid of the symptoms, maybe not even all of them but at least the ones that bother us most. Thus we look at illness from our mechanistic viewpoint - a breakdown in the machine, which must be fixed as quickly as possible.

Sickness and troubles are a normal part of life, not necessarily as obstacles but as indicators of where we are on our path. They may even be beacons showing the way through our inner night. We need to move away from thinking we are either ill or well, and realize that what happens to us represents the stages of a process, the process of life. Rejecting part of what happens to us amounts to a separation from a part of our life.

Illness can be seen as an invitation to become aware of our weak points, so that we can work out how to strengthen them and widen our understanding of ourselves. Ultimately it is in overcoming the hurdles that life puts in our path, not in dodging round them, that we discover our true strength.

EXERCISE 4: *WHAT DOES ILLNESS MEAN TO YOU?*
Consider these questions to evaluate the role of illness in your life.

What meaning does it have to you to be ill?
What place does illness have in life, as you see it? Why does illness exist?
In what way does the existence of illness affect your view of life?

What feelings does illness stir in you? Insecurity, incomprehension, fear, vulnerability, feeling threatened or that it is unfair, despair, ...

What positive aspects of illness can you find?

The body's way of claiming attention

Many of our inner struggles arise from a pull in different directions between the ego and the higher self (see page 43). The ego, which is linked with the physical, emotional, and mental bodies, holds our familiar patterns of thinking and acting. The causal and spiritual bodies are linked with the higher self - our true nature and source of our inner wisdom - which encourages our true gifts and qualities to show themselves. If we do not willingly pay attention to this struggle then our system may create physical symptoms and illnesses to make us take notice.

Other illnesses can be seen as the battle between nature and the collective human ego,

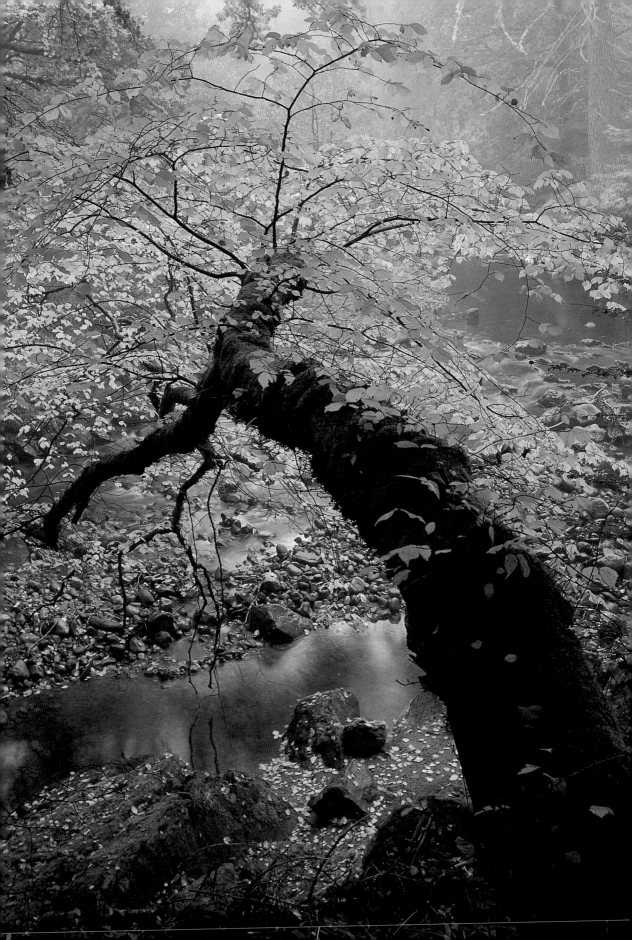

such as those resulting from pollution, from our treatment of animals (mad cow disease, myxamatosis), or from our supermarket attitude to medicine: dependence on psychotropic drugs, or infections resistant to antibiotics.

A crisis leading to personal growth

When you are in acute pain of body or soul, it may be hard to accept that it is all for the sake of your personal growth. However, it can be helpful to think about a crisis from this point of view in a calmer moment. By "crisis" we mean any acute disturbance in your life. Examples of physical crises are a pain, a malfunction in an organ or one of the body's systems, a fever, or an injury. Mental crises include all stressful situations that disturb the tranquillity of life. These range from the stress you experience when you meet a stranger, which usually passes in a matter of seconds, through longer lasting reactions to major life events, such as losing your job or starting a new one, bereavement, divorce, or moving house.

The exercises on this page will help you to evaluate past crises in your life and recognize that they may have had positive effects.

EXERCISE 5:
MY PERSONAL EVOLUTION

This exercise helps you see how coping with crises has helped you along your own personal path to self-awareness.

During which period of my life have I evolved the most?
Which situations have provoked the most change?

For each of these situations:
How did I regard the problem when it came up?
What qualities did I call on to cope with it?
With hindsight, how do these events look to me now?
What qualities did the situation teach me and bring out in me?

EXERCISE 6:
MY MOST RECENT CRISIS

Considering a crisis you have been through provides an opportunity for discovering that it was not only a negative or destructive experience.

What effects has it had in my life?
What did it make clear to me?
In what way has it enriched me?
What lasting benefits has it brought into my life?

51

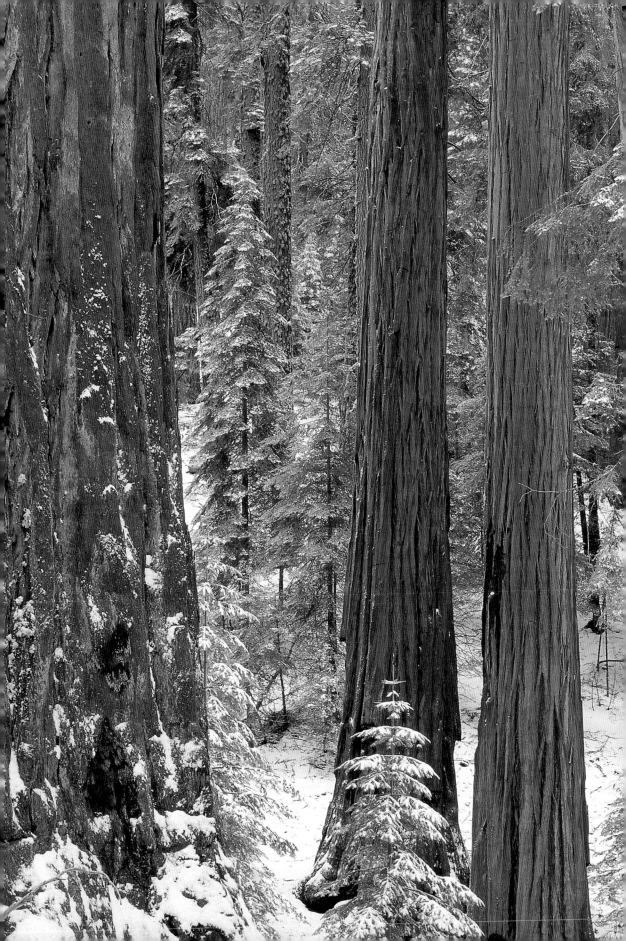

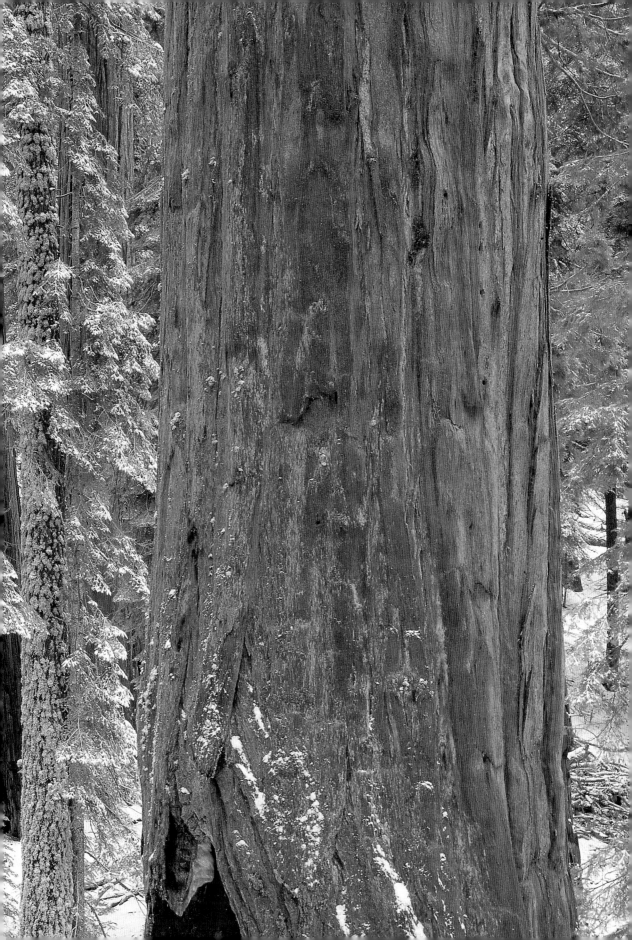

The seven stages of healing

The development of an illness or problem follows a common sequence, whether it's a physical illness, a personal crisis, or a problem in a relationship. This same sequence is set in motion by any crisis, from a meeting with a stranger, when the stages flash by in seconds, to more long-term problems, such as the effort to come to terms with a lack of parental love and attention, where one stage may last several years. The seven stages of this sequence are described right and on pages 56-60.

If you were to look at a view through a tube, you would see only a tiny part of it, but you would think this tiny part was the whole picture. Then if you looked through a wider tube, you would see new parts of the scene, which then make a new whole. In the same way we perceive our problems according to the width of our own "tube", that is, the level of our consciousness at a given time. So as our awareness broadens, other aspects of the problem become visible and our picture of the problem becomes more complete.

This expansion of awareness is a natural process. If you consider the fundamental questions about life, such as "Who am I?" or "What is God?" you will see that the answers you bring to them now are not the same as those you would have given five, ten, or twenty years ago. Your response evolves over time, according to who you were and who you have become as a result of your life experiences - in other words, in relation to the opening of your consciousness.

Evolution to higher levels of consciousness is not linear but in an ascending spiral (see facing page). You may revisit old problems again at each level in the spiral, but even if it is the same old issue, your view of it has changed because you have been making steady upward progress, and you will now have new means at your disposal for finding a new answer to it.

THE SEVEN STAGES

❶ The problem appears.

❷ The ego resists - my first reaction to the problem.

❸ Seeing what the problem reveals - I begin to adapt.

❹ Experimenting with another attitude - I think again and try a new way of behaving in the situation.

❺ New qualities come in - my new attitude frees qualities within me.

❻ The new attitude changes the situation - I feel release.

❼ I integrate what has happened.

Stages 1-4:
the response of the ego

Stages 5-7:
freeing the higher self

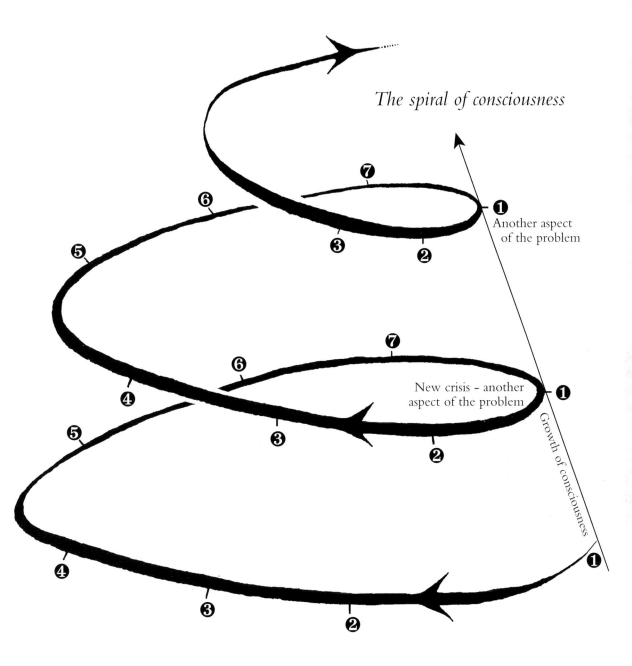

The spiral of consciousness

① Another aspect
of the problem

New crisis - another
aspect of the problem ①

Growth of consciousness

At each level of the spiral you work through the seven stages until you reach a deeper understanding, when you "jump" up to the next level. This jump represents a change in attitude to the problem. You may then meet another aspect of the same problem again at this new level. This does not mean that you have moved backward, but that your consciousness has grown and broadened, which allows you to access a new understanding.

The process that leads to long-term healing, as opposed to the temporary suppression of symptoms, has two complementary aspects: clarifying the ego and freeing your capacity for self-healing by letting the higher self emerge. It is like being in a room with dirty windows and wanting to see the sun. The obvious first step is to clean the windows, and then the sun, which is always shining, can come flooding in.

S T A G E 1 : *THE PROBLEM APPEARS*

The healing process begins when I notice the problem in its present form. It may have been there for some time without my noticing it. An illness can have an incubation period of several days, or even years, and it is only when it begins to make us suffer that we start the process of adaptation. And it is possible to live for many years in the grip of an emotional problem without realizing it. For example, if I am unable to cope with others' authority, and end up in a confrontation every time I am stopped by the police or go through customs, it might be years before I realize that I am unconsciously creating these situations for myself.

S T A G E 2 : *THE EGO RESISTS*

I react to the situation with symptoms or feelings that show there is a struggle going on inside. The body fights the invading germs or infection, creating a fever, or the emotions fight against the person or situation that has triggered the crisis. Most of the time the ego is caught up in feelings and fixed ideas which create a fog that blinds us to what is really happening. The feelings triggered in us by our relationships with the opposite sex, the family, money, success, power, violence, prevent us from seeing things clearly. As soon as we get into a situation involving these issues we are so busy reacting to disguise our distress that we completely lose our objectivity. Our habitual thought patterns can complicate things for us in the same way. Some are so deeply ingrained that it never occurs to us to question them.

In the confrontation between the ego and the cause of the trouble, the emotional and mental bodies work together to resist the new situation. Your thoughts and feelings rush in all directions to find a way out. In stage 2 you are stuck in your idea of how you think you are, which guides your thoughts and feelings. Exercise 7 (see facing page) gives you practice in freeing yourself from these fixed patterns so that you can move on to stage 3.

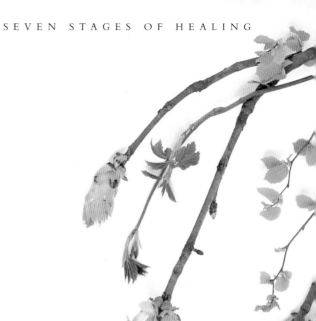
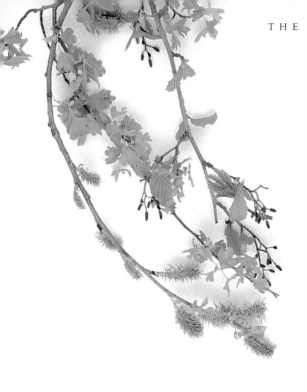

EXERCISE 7: *RELEASING SUPERFLUOUS THOUGHTS*

This practical technique helps you break out of your rigid ideas, giving you the mental space to see what a problem reveals.

Find a flower in bloom, settle yourself comfortably in front of it and explore into its very depths. Immediately a thought will spring to mind, probably a judgement such as, "isn't it fragile", or "how pretty", or whatever. As soon as you are aware of the thought, acknowledge that it is interrupting the exchange between you and the flower, and however correct or poetic the thought may be, let it go. Another one will pop up, so let that go too, and allow your thoughts to peel away like the layers of an onion. Suddenly, when the thoughts are all gone, you will experience the flower as it is - and what a surprise this can be.

STAGE 3: *SEEING WHAT THE PROBLEM REVEALS*

In spite of the problem, life must go on and I realize I have to pull myself together and not allow myself to be overwhelmed. At this point the ego usually makes some compromises to limit the suffering and loss of power in the face of the problem. Whatever your thoughts or emotions aroused by what is happening, you have to accept responsibility for them, especially if they are not very praiseworthy. You also have to accept responsibility for decisions you make, such as rejecting the person or the situation causing you the problem, and the consequences of such decisions.

At this stage the situation is changing but the problem is not really solved; it may be displaced to a slightly different context or replaced by another version of the same issue. For example, if a woman leaves her violent alcoholic husband, at first she feels relief because she is no longer in danger from his violence. But after a while she may begin to feel lonely and become depressed. She has moved from one problem scenario to another.

In a physical illness, this is the stage where the fever reaches a plateau, the temperature stops rising and is high, but stable.

STAGE 4: *EXPERIMENTING WITH ANOTHER ATTITUDE*

This stage is a major turning point, where the ego is cleared, allowing the higher self to emerge. In order to facilitate this you need to look at your past behaviour, to see how it has contributed to your present situation. Do you feel you have had a hand in creating this situation? How does it relate to other problems in your life? What is your life trying to teach you at the moment? What changes in your behaviour would change the situation?

From this you may be able to identify specific behaviour that you can try to change: for example, being less critical of your partner's untidiness, or making sure you allow yourself time for relaxation. You can then try out this new attitude next time the situation arises. This experimentation with a new behaviour initially requires conscious effort, but gradually you begin to adopt the new pattern.

In the example of the fever, once you have reached this stage of adopting a new attitude, your temperature will begin to fall.

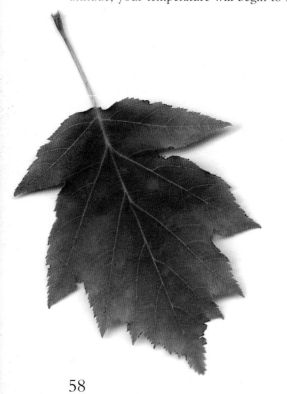

EXERCISE 8: *ADOPTING A DIFFERENT ATTITUDE*

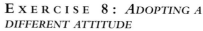

The way we formulate our problems often reveals where we are putting the blame for them. Try turning around your usual formula and see what happens.

❶ Find a sentence that sums up your problem. For example, "My partner is impossible: he has no respect for me and never takes any notice of what I want."

❷ Now turn your sentence around, replacing each reference to the other by referring to yourself. The sentence becomes "I don't manage to make myself respected by my partner and I find it hard to say clearly what I want."

As long as you put all the blame for the situation on the other person you are powerless. By looking at your own part in it you can see what you can do to change things. Thus out of a problem comes an opportunity to grow.

STAGE 5: *NEW QUALITIES COME IN*

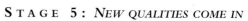

The new behaviour that I consciously adopted in stage 4 has become a part of me, allowing new qualities to develop. It no longer takes a conscious effort and I bring these qualities to every situation, for example being more loving, more tolerant, less critical.

This process gives you a new point of view, which was activated by the desire to transform the situation by becoming more responsible and more loving. The first panic of feeling threatened has given way to a desire to solve the problem, so it is easier to be objective instead of getting carried away in reactions.

In the case of the physical illness, your body is starting to recover. It has overcome the infection and the fever decreases.

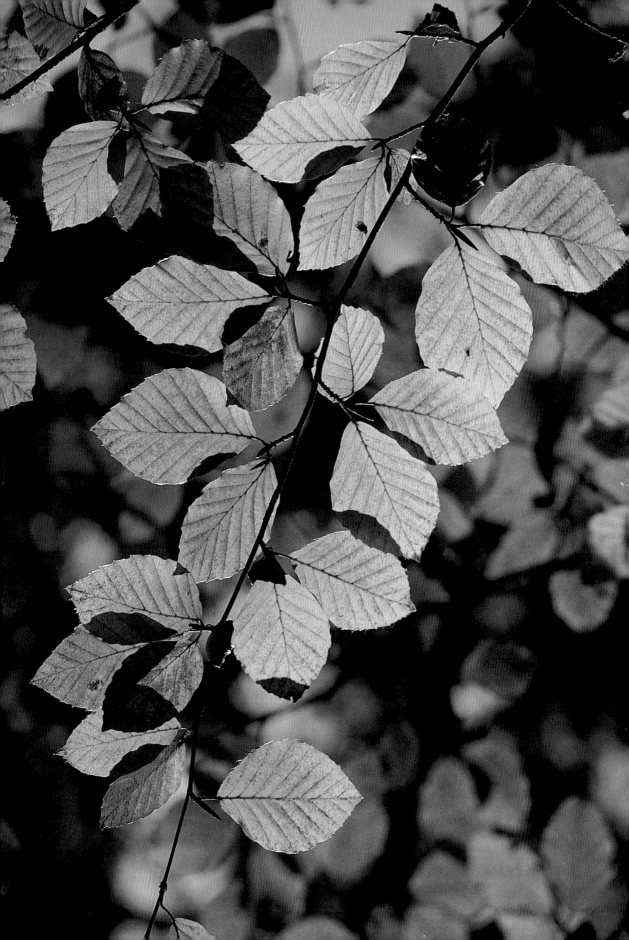

STAGE 6: *THE NEW ATTITUDE CHANGES THE SITUATION*

The changes you have made in your own behaviour pattern, and the qualities this has released, create a new situation. For example, if a man cannot deal with aggressive behaviour in others, he may be assertive and challenge aggression wherever he meets it. But his behaviour will then tend to bring out the aggressive side of other people. If he can solve his inner problem, he will no longer be in confrontation with the problem, and he will be able to see others as they truly are.

In mastering a problem you create an inner freedom, which leaves you feeling lighter and comfortable with yourself. This is the stage in a physical illness when you begin to feel better - the fever has almost gone.

STAGE 7: *I INTEGRATE WHAT HAS HAPPENED*

This is the stage of convalescence, when I have got over the illness but still need to take care to avoid a relapse. This phase is just as important for a mental or emotional problem as it is for a physical one. Sometimes when there has been a major shift in our way of being, the ego gets nervous and may take some time to get used to the new situation. It is important to pay attention to new energy patterns and make sure that they don't slip back into old grooves (see Exercise 9 below). Also be aware of others involved in the situation, for when real change happens it releases new energies that affect all concerned.

EXAMPLE: *THE SEVEN STAGES IN A PHYSICAL PROBLEM*

Stage 1: I feel hot/cold/stiff.
Stage 2: On no! I won't be able to go to Carole's birthday party.
Stage 3: I'll go to bed with a hot water bottle and sweat it out.
Stage 4: What has happened to me? I'd better take a bit more care of myself. I've been burning the candle at both ends, getting over-tired, ignoring my limits. Maybe my mother's illness and that trouble at work have taken more out of me than I realized.
Stage 5: I'll stay in bed and take some time for myself. I'll have a real rest and fast for a day.
Stage 6: My body feels a bit better, the illness is losing its grip and the fever is almost gone.
Stage 7: I feel completely better. From now on I'll pay more attention to myself, to my own kind of energy, to my own rhythms, my limits, and my needs.

EXERCISE 9: *SELF-ANALYSIS*

This exercise helps you evaluate your experiences and the benefits you have gained from a crisis.

Find a space to be quiet and take time to consider how the situation arose.

What was going on in your life in the period just before the problem or symptoms became obvious?
What feelings did these events stir up?
What experiences from the past did they remind you of?
What weakness or lack of power did this evoke?
What were you not paying enough attention to before the crisis became obvious?

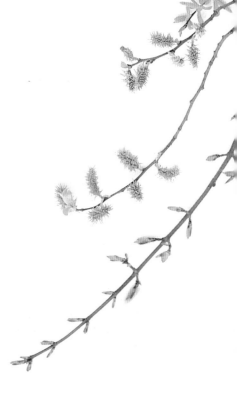

It is all too easy to think that being sick is the opposite of being well - that we are either in one state or the other, either in a crisis or everything is fine. If we remain stuck in this polarized attitude we miss out on learning all that an illness or problem can teach us about our own personal growth and enlarging our repertoire of behaviour. Realizing that an illness follows a specific sequence helps us out of this trap.

When you next face an illness or a difficult situation, take time to consider which stage you are at in the process, and you will come closer to the heart of the matter. Notice too when one stage shifts into another - this will enable you to see how far you have come since the problem started and to have a realistic idea of the stages still to go through. This is one way of keeping hold of the power that is lost if you hope to attain an idealized state of being "well" that does not seem to have any connection with where you are now.

When the time is ripe you will heal yourself, or rather your energy bodies will align themselves in a way that allows them to get in touch with the central knot of the problem. The tangles release, and you are healed of the distortions caused at every level, including the physical symptoms.

This approach means having the faith and the confidence to let the process unravel. An illness or a personal crisis is actually an invitation to us to move forward in life. And in the end we come to realize that whatever the problem, it mirrors something inside us, and it is in our inner world that we can find its resolution. The problems we encounter lead us to an encounter with ourselves.

In Chapter 3 you will see how encounters with trees will help you develop the attitudes you need in order to be fully present at this meeting with yourself.

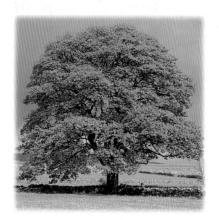

Chapter 3

Expanding our perception of trees

What can be more majestic than a great tree in its prime, or more moving than a fruit tree snowed under by its spring blossom? Have you ever sensed as you gaze at its beauty, the mysterious life that makes this tree what it is? But how can you make contact with this living tree? Our usual ways of thinking and looking at the world aren't much help, and only lead to frustration and doubt. In the last chapter we discovered that taking a fresh look at illness gives us a fresh perspective on ourselves, and in the same way, exploring ways of making contact with trees will reveal much about them and also about ourselves.

This chapter leads you along this path of exploration, through exercises to be done outside among the trees. As these bring you closer to the mystery of the tree they also bring you into closer contact with the mystery of yourself. You have already experienced the challenge of opening yourself to a new understanding of illness; now the challenge is to open yourself to a new understanding of the living being that is the tree. You will find that the tree offers you gifts that make this opening worthwhile.

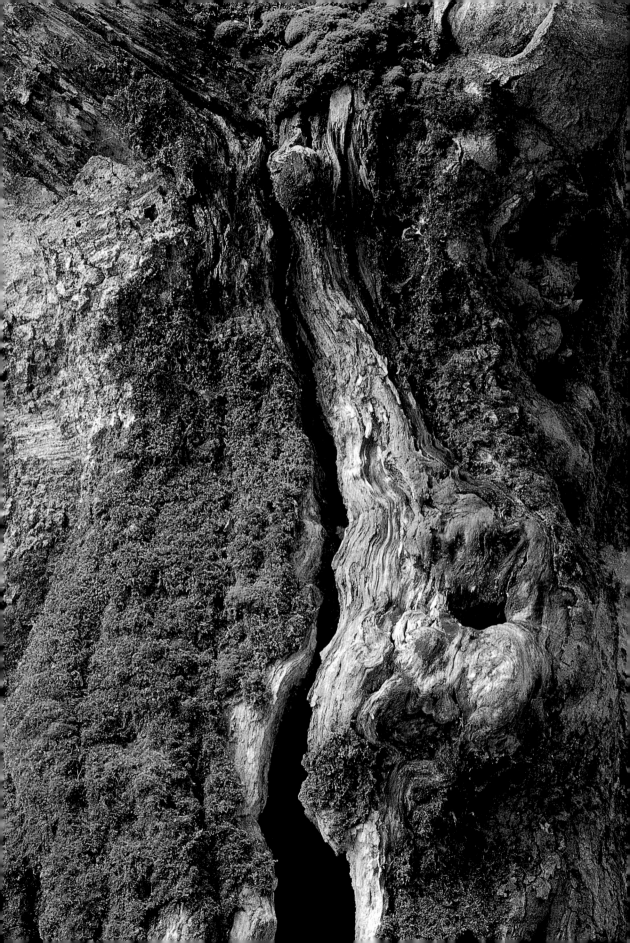

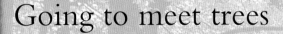

Going to meet trees

You may be lucky enough to live in a place where trees are part of your everyday surroundings. But how often do you really see them and appreciate their presence?

We take trees so much for granted. But within their familiar shapes we can glimpse the mystery of the living power of nature, a power our present way of life does little to nourish. Maybe it is our unconscious hunger to reconnect with this power that is making us more aware of the presence of trees among us. You may have already felt the touch of this mystery. The exercises that follow go further in exploring what happens when you pay full attention to a tree.

EXERCISE 10:
A WALKING MEDITATION

This exercise will help you observe yourself when you go for a walk in the woods or the forest. The state of mind in which you walk will condition the experiences you have, and the potential effects of the later exercises.
We often walk through the woods in the same attitude as through the supermarket. The mind is in fact going over what we did yesterday or just now and planning what we are going to do tomorrow, and the present slips by unnoticed.

❶ First come into the present. Listen to your own breathing, feel the earth beneath your feet, and get the sense of how you are balanced.

❷ Listen to how your mind is organizing your walk: "I won't go that way, there are some brambles ... over there it's muddy, so I won't go that way ..."
We are always giving ourselves instructions, imposing limits and forbidding things, when the joy of life is to release ourselves from limitations. When you surprise yourself doing it, don't judge yourself, just smile. Then carry on and follow wherever your feet want to take you.

It is wonderful to realise that you are in a place you would never have found if you had only done what your mind was telling you or followed your old habits. It means you have let yourself be guided by your intuition - your higher self.

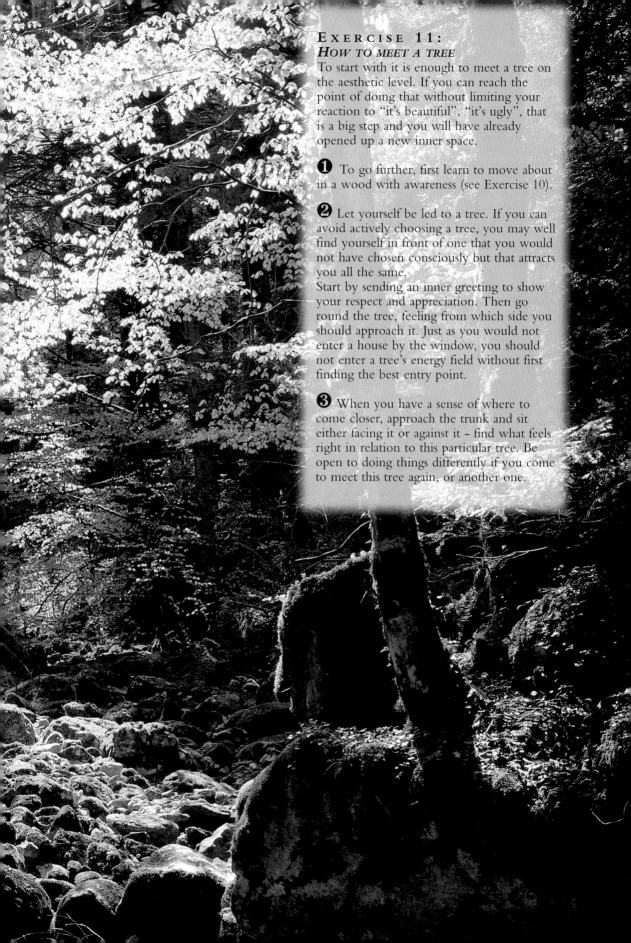

EXERCISE 11:
HOW TO MEET A TREE

To start with it is enough to meet a tree on the aesthetic level. If you can reach the point of doing that without limiting your reaction to "it's beautiful", "it's ugly", that is a big step and you will have already opened up a new inner space.

❶ To go further, first learn to move about in a wood with awareness (see Exercise 10).

❷ Let yourself be led to a tree. If you can avoid actively choosing a tree, you may well find yourself in front of one that you would not have chosen consciously but that attracts you all the same.

Start by sending an inner greeting to show your respect and appreciation. Then go round the tree, feeling from which side you should approach it. Just as you would not enter a house by the window, you should not enter a tree's energy field without first finding the best entry point.

❸ When you have a sense of where to come closer, approach the trunk and sit either facing it or against it – find what feels right in relation to this particular tree. Be open to doing things differently if you come to meet this tree again, or another one.

Using the five senses

Do not expect that your very first experiences of contact with a tree will be mind-blowing. It is a mistake to try to bypass the natural stages of your own development or to delude yourself with fantasies of transcendence. To keep your feet on the ground and stay in contact with physical reality, use your five senses. They can be the doorways to a perception of reality wider than you have dreamed of. It is the use we make of our senses and the way that our mind processes the wealth of information that they supply to it, that limits our sensory perceptions. But we know that beyond ordinary sight is clairvoyance, beyond everyday hearing is clairaudience, beyond ordinary touching there is another level of sensitivity. So let us open these doors a little wider.

Sight

We each have in our brain a stock of images accumulated over a lifetime, and when we see something our optical system identifies it by checking it against the images already in store. There is a parallel with the saying of Plato that we do not so much invent as reinvent the world – in other words, we refer everything back to what we already know. The result is that we don't really see things: we stop looking as soon as the mind has identified them, so it is difficult for us to discover anything genuinely new.

In our culture the faculty of sight is constantly bombarded, by traffic signals, by advertising, by the television that is the intermediary in so much of our experience of the world, by the computer screen we have to concentrate on for work, as well as by the words and pictures in an ocean of printed matter. On account of this over-use of our sight, the brain systems relating to it are very active and the neurone pathways carrying visual information are well worn, so it may be useful to extend our experience of sight.

EXERCISE 12:
GOING BEYOND OUR LIMITS

The habits of perception that govern our sight, so that we look at things without really seeing them, also limit our capacity to perceive in other ways. Our mental habits are just as limiting, so here is a chance to explore and go beyond them.

❶ Sit down somewhere quiet in the woods and look at the scene in a general way, not stopping for details but letting your gaze move all around you. You will notice that your field of vision has a radius of perhaps twenty metres (sixty-five feet), and that it is bounded by a first screen of trees. Concentrate on the trees that stop you seeing further, and then look for the spaces between the branches and leaves through which you can glimpse the trees beyond. As you adjust you realize the first row is no longer a barrier, and that you are aware of a much bigger space.

❷ This brings you to the second screen of trees. As with the first one, don't let it stop you but look further still between its branches to the trees beyond. Soon that barrier too dissolves, and a much wider reality opens up around you. Don't rush the process, or try right away to see as far as possible, because if you jump from the foreground to the far distance you'll miss all that the in-between stages can offer as a model for expanding your awareness.

Noticing how you travel is more important than seeing how far you can go.

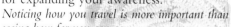

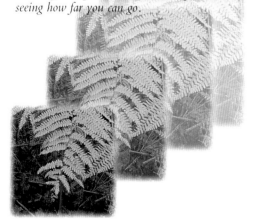

EXERCISE 13:
THE SURPRISE OF THE FAMILIAR

What you have been trying out with the very big, you can also do with the very small. In contrast to the last exercise where the view is panoramic, in this one you focus your vision on the very small.

❶ Look down at a patch of grass from your full height. This gives you an instant picture of it. Now slow down and look more closely, and you'll see lots of things you didn't notice at first: dead wood, new shoots, lumps of earth, or bits and pieces chewed by insects.

❷ Next bend down and get closer, and you discover even more details in what you think you have seen. The more attention you give, the more details you discover and the more surprises you get. Each time you stop and say "Well, now I've seen everything", take a deep breath and say instead, "What am I going to discover next?"

If you do this exercise properly you can go on discovering things for hours. The results can be amazing. Treat it like a meditation and accept the meaning it has for your consciousness.

Hearing

Our hearing provides more spatial information than does our sight, but we scarcely notice the physiological process by which it works.

When you go into the woods, don't just stop at saying, "How wonderful the silence is!" because in a wood it isn't ever silent, it is just that there is no sound actually intruding on your ear. To get to know the forest, listen! Let your ears open to the sounds that are there.

Observe closely in what part of your body you hear a particular sound. You will come to realise that you can hear through other places than your ears, which turns our accepted ideas upside down but opens a gateway into new realms of understanding the world we live in.

CASE STUDY

Anne Catherine, a deaf woman, took off her hearing aid for this exercise in one of my workshops. We were all astonished by the finesse of her hearing perception, though she couldn't say where she heard the sounds.

EXERCISE 14:
LISTENING TO THE TREES

This is an exercise for refining your hearing and learning to open your ears to sounds instead of ignoring them until they invade.

❶ Find a place in the woods that inspires you, and settle down. Open your hearing first of all to the sounds you hear without effort - the birds singing, the wind blowing, the branches creaking - and then to all the others, down to the very smallest.

❷ Then experiment a little. Put your ear to the ground, as the Amerindians do, to find out if anything is approaching. Put your ear to the trunk of a tree, and don't just stop at, "Yes, I can hear something". Stay with it, see how this sound affects you. What quality does it have? Where does it resonate in your body? And the sound itself, what does it do? Listen how it gets louder or quieter, or mingles with other sounds.
You may not notice much detail at first, but as you repeat the exercise you will be surprised at what happens.

Touch

This is a sense that is ignored for two reasons: for one it has become taboo in our culture, and for another it does not lend itself to mass communication as do sight and hearing. In fact it is often the shadow sister of the faculty of sight; before touching anything we establish visual contact with it, and thus make up a mental image of it first. So if you wish to discover trees by touch, you must first close your eyes. We do not touch only with our hands: the whole body can experience touch, and our feet are in constant touch with the earth. The way we encounter the ground beneath us through our feet is something we pay little attention to, or process first through our eyes.

The exercise (left) calls on several aspects of our experience: the sense of touch, of balance, of movement, how we handle our fears, and a host of other things. It covers so much that we could spend days afterward digesting what it has taught us.

EXERCISE 15:
THE BLIND PERSON AND THE GUARDIAN ANGEL
This is an exercise to do in pairs.

❶ One person, who is blindfolded, goes for a walk among the trees, accompanied by the other as guardian angel, who keeps their eyes open. Agree a time at the beginning – 20 minutes is about right. The guardian angel should keep an eye on the time so they can warn their partner a few minutes before the end, giving them time to regain their ordinary functioning.

❷ The blindfolded partner goes where they want, stops, moves on, touches things, tries to keep their balance. The guardian angel is not there to stop them getting into trouble, only to keep an eye out for real danger. When the other gets into difficulties, the guardian observes how they react. Sometimes they'll extract themselves from a dense thicket as if it were hardly there, or get tangled up in a nothing of a bush as if in the Amazon jungle.

❸ It is important to remain silent. The guardian angel can warn the other of danger by a touch on the arm or shoulder. The silence is revealing too for the guardian, making them aware of how they give help, of their fears for other people, how they interfere in what others are doing.

Smell

We generally notice only those smells that are intrusive. However it is not our sense of smell that is limited, but the way that the mind processes the information it receives from the sensitive membranes in the nasal passages. As with our other senses, we can improve our perceptions and thus our ability to distinguish the subtle smells of the woods, which reveal themselves only to those who go to meet them.

Certain smells have a vibratory level so subtle that they can carry you to higher levels of consciousness which transcend the realities perceived by our ordinary senses. Maybe there is a faculty of "clair-olfaction" - a sense beyond the ordinary sense of smell.

The two stages of Exercise 16 each activate one side of the brain to refine the sense of smell. You can do them in either order, but it is more effective to do them on separate occasions rather than one after the other.

EXERCISE 16:

LEARNING TO SMELL

If you try to discover the smells around you with a few sniffs, like a dog following a scent, you will soon be hyperventilating. For both the exercises use the following technique.

Don't be in any hurry; breathe normally and calmly. As you breathe in, bring your attention into your nose, and notice the smell. Then let the breath out again as usual, waiting for the next inbreath to bring you the smell again.

Identify the smells if you can: sweet, bitter, acrid, woody, or flowery. Probably others you cannot identify will surprise you, but don't let the surprise stop you savouring them and finding which ones you enjoy.

❶ Let your curiosity lead you to explore the smells of a tree trunk, its buds, the fallen leaves, the soil. In this exercise you go to look for the smells.
This is an analytic perception that activates the left side of the brain.

❷ Take time to notice the smells that come to you. Settle yourself comfortably, at the foot of a tree for example, and smell the air, noticing how one smell is wafted after another, like clouds drifting across the sky.
This is a more global perception that activates the right side of the brain.

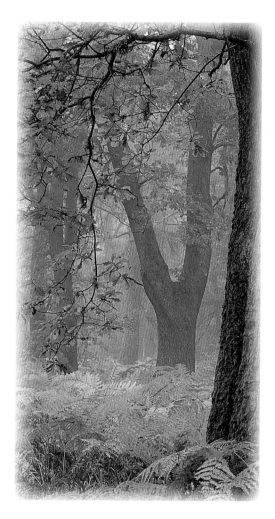

Taste

Our capacity for taste is often stunted by the habit of immediately chewing and swallowing whatever we put in our mouths, without taking the time to taste it. You may like to try tasting the buds, sap, flowers, or fruit of certain trees, but caution is needed, as some of these may be poisonous. Do not experiment unless you are certain that what you are tasting is safe.

EXERCISE 17:
EXPANDING THE PERCEPTION OF TASTE
Use this technique to become aware of the subtle tastes and flavours of parts of a tree. Only taste the bud, leaf, flower, sap, or any other part of the tree if you are absolutely certain that it is not poisonous or harmful.

❶ Whatever part of the tree you choose, chew it first and remind yourself that you are not going to swallow it. This switches off your usual reflex. Chew slowly and notice how your mouth responds, whether the saliva comes readily or not.

❷ Pause now and again to notice the tastes that are there, and to see if they are different from at first.
When you have had enough, spit it all out and check again what taste is present.
Does it last or fade quickly?
What reactions do these tastes set off in your body? Resistance, pleasure, calm, excitement, ...

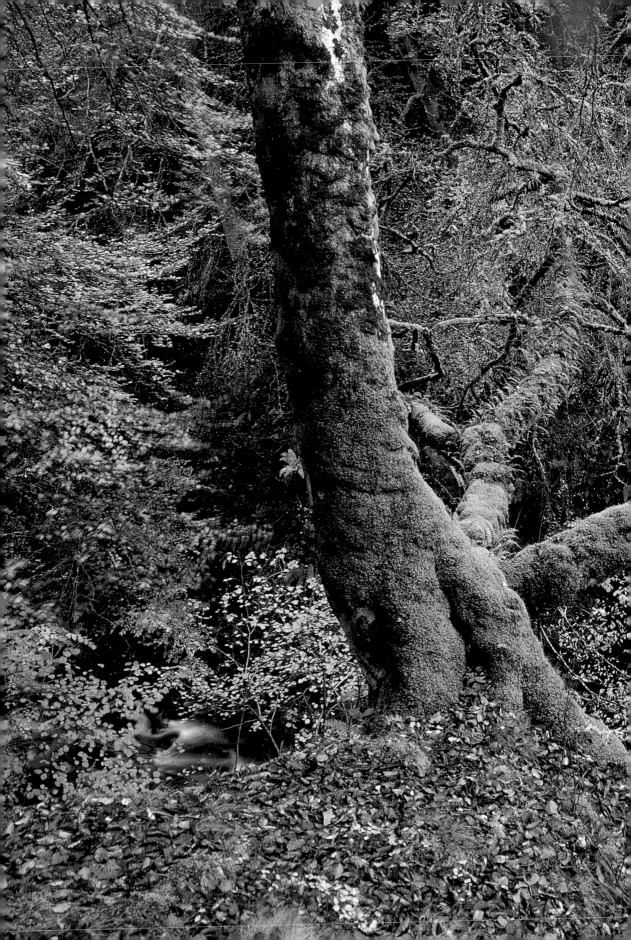

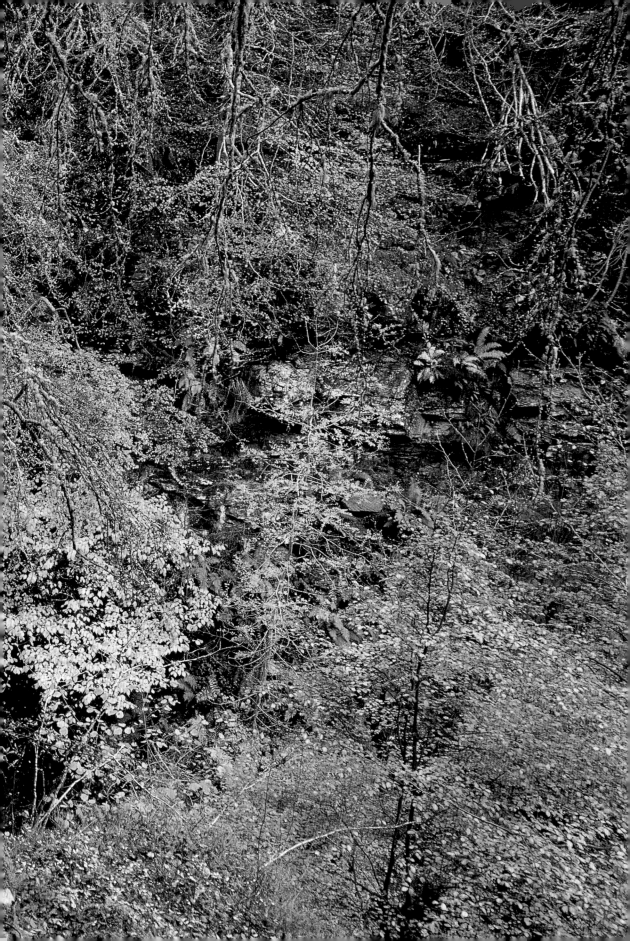

Moving from perception to awareness

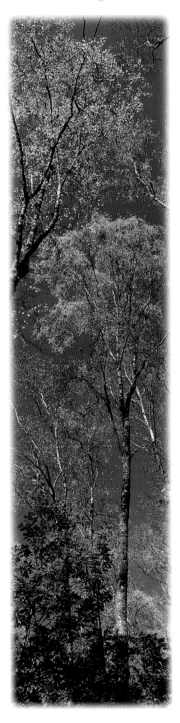

From the exercises so far you will have found out something new about trees, and maybe begun to see them differently. Normally we look at a tree as something exterior to ourselves. We use what our senses tell us to construct a whole world "out there", but in fact we are not separate from it, since what we see often affects our inner state. We look at something beautiful which puts us in a state of inner grace; we sense a splendour in what is before us and are filled with gratitude.

Much of this happens without our realizing it, and it is the same with our other senses. What we hear or smell also has a resonance within us, which will differ from one person to another. Often two people involved in the same situation will see the same thing but respond in completely different ways, to the point where you wonder if they actually saw the same incident. This is the interface between our senses and our consciousness; what our senses perceive is filtered according to how open and aware we are prepared to be. The next exercises help you to increase your awareness even further, through movement, sound, and breathing.

Movement

When you see someone whose body is stiff you can imagine how stiff they are also in their patterns of thought. Restricted movements often indicate someone trying to create a false image of them-selves, while someone who is imprecise and lethargic in their movements is probably not making much effort at all. The kinds of movement people make often reveal a lot about their dynamic in life, or lack of it. Although we think of trees as stationary, they have their own individual ways of moving in the wind, so watching a tree's move-ments is good preparation for understanding its energetic qualities. Trees also have their own more subtle movements, which it is possible to explore.

DISCOVERING HOW A TREE MOVES

To discover all there is to learn from a tree's movements you need to observe it closely and take time to tune in with it.

❶ Find a tree that appeals to you, and stand in front of it with your hands on each side of the trunk, arms stretched out but relaxed. Tilt your head back so that you can watch the movements of the branches and leaves.

❷ Let your attention widen to take in the tree as a whole, and sense how it is moving. Let your body sway with it, and gradually you will begin to share in the movement and feel it in your own body. When you can feel this, close your eyes, keeping your hands on the trunk, and let the movement continue. If you are used to dancing or expressing through your body, do not hesitate to release your hold on the trunk and create a dance in resonance with the subtle movements of the tree.

A word of caution: if you stay for a while with your head tilted back you may feel dizzy, because this position restricts some of the blood vessels in the neck. If this occurs, simply straighten your neck and relax until the dizziness passes.

EXERCISE 19:
USING YOUR VOICE

The idea of this exercise is to find the sound that will create a dynamic contact with the tree by putting you in resonance with it.

❶ Choose a tree and stand in front of it. Staying in contact with this tree by touch and with your thoughts, try out different notes until you find the one that is easiest to produce. You'll know when it is the right one because with no extra effort on your part it will come out twice as loud as the others. Then pause to hear the reply or the echo that the tree sends back.

❷ Make another sound on a different note, guided by the response you have heard. Listen again for the echo, then make another sound, and so on.

Gradually the gaps of silence shorten and, if you can silence your mental critic, you find yourself carried into a song that brings into form an aspect of the energy of the tree. Then you are truly in communication with the tree, and your song expresses the inspiration it is sending you.

Sound

Another gateway into a deeper perception of the tree is through using your voice. In Exercise 18 you may have realized that even when a tree is not moving in the wind there are still subtle movements inside it: the signs of its life rhythms. So subtle are they that your own movements feel too clumsy to match them, and you may find you can echo these rhythms more closely through using sound (Exercise 19). Your voice can create such a wide range of frequencies that you are bound to find some that resonate with the tree. It may feel awkward at first, but it is worth persevering to experience the deep contact with the tree.

Breathing

Have you ever experienced meeting someone with whom you felt an almost instantaneous rapport? You quickly feel at ease with this person and on the same wavelength, and your body language and even your breathing rhythm adapt itself to theirs. Conversely, when you meet somebody stressed out your breathing becomes faster and shallower as you pick up their vibrations.

With practice you can become aware of these responses, which usually go unnoticed, and you'll understand much more of what goes on at every level in relating to other people. The same sort of reactions occur when you come close to a tree. Of course the senses are all involved - you can see and hear and smell and touch the tree - and at the same time a more subtle interaction is taking place. Under one tree you may feel it is easy to rest; another may be stimulating; and another you may want to get away from. This is because trees also have their individuality, and as with people, some are easier to feel in harmony with than others. What happens to your breathing is a good indication of how you are responding to the encounter. Exercise 20 gives you practice in observing your responses.

Experiencing this exchange with the tree through breathing takes us toward the limit of what we can feel through our sensory mechanisms. If you go into it fully you enter into a real exchange between yourself and the tree.

EXERCISE 20: *BREATHING IN THE PRESENCE OF A TREE*

To discover how the exchange with the tree affects your breathing, you need first to notice each part of your normal breathing pattern. Don't try to change it; just pay attention to how it moves naturally.

❶ Sit somewhere quietly and observe where your breathing is coming from: your belly, your diaphragm area, your throat? Then observe its amplitude: how much you fill up with each inbreath and how much you let out with the outbreath. Are there parts of your body that don't fill up?

❷ Now observe the rhythm: is it rapid, regular, uneven? Then observe its quality: peaceful, energetic, assured, anxious?

❸ Now that you have a sense of your usual breathing pattern, find a tree that appeals to you and make yourself comfortable against it. Relax.
Notice how you are breathing now. Check the same points: where it starts from, its amplitude, its rhythm, and its quality. Have any of these factors changed?
Take as much time as you need. Then when you feel you have done enough, thank the tree and go to another one. Repeat the experiment, and see what, if anything, is different this time.

By the time you have tried this exercise with several trees of different kinds and different sizes you will have become more sensitive. You will then be able to choose a tree that will help you feel more calm or more energized, or whatever it is that you need.

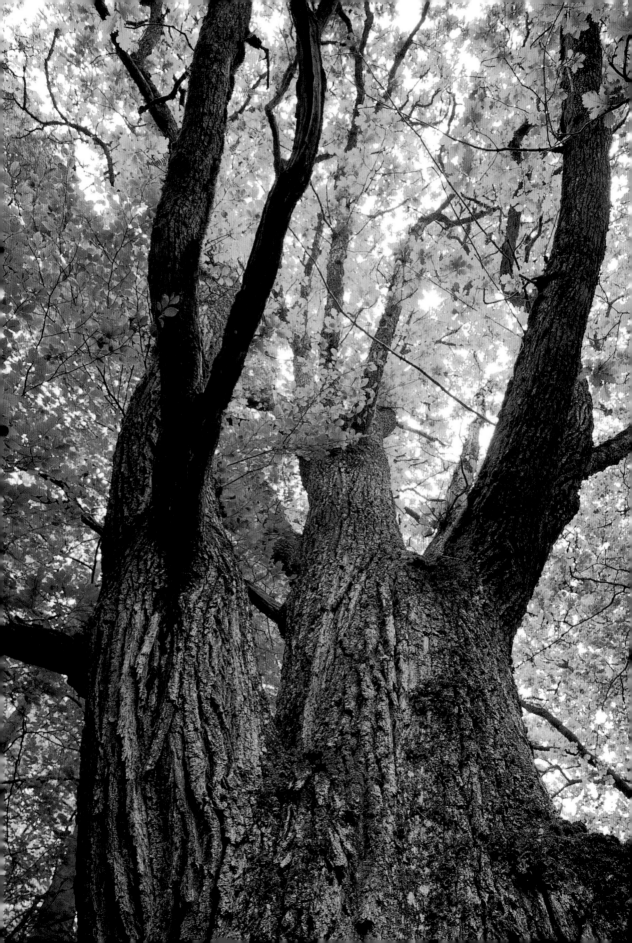

Discovering the energy field of a tree

To understand how something as personal as your breathing pattern can be affected by the presence of a tree, we need to consider what happens at an energetic level. Each tree (and indeed every living being) has an energy field that radiates from it, in the same way as an energy field radiates from a person (see Chapter 2). When you encounter a tree your energy field reacts and adapts to its energy field. This adaptation may be too subtle to notice at first, but you respond with a series of shifts in your metabolism, your thoughts, and your feelings. Since the tree has none of the fluctuations of a human ego, its energy pattern is more constant than ours and it provides a tool for understanding our own patterns of response.

A tree's energy field has layers which express different rhythms. With practice most people can sense these differences, although not everyone feels exactly the same thing. In most trees the basic rhythm is the annual cycle of growth and renewal through the seasons. Then there is the rhythm of day and night, which peaks at the moment of sunrise. Each tree also has its own more obscure rhythms which create its particular quality.

One way to refine your capacity to hear these rhythms is to listen to your breathing pattern. With practice you'll be able to tell if your breathing is peaceful, anxious, nervous, holding back, or free. Once you can "hear" well enough to do this you can listen for the rhythms in a tree in the same way as you listen to your own breathing.

The exercises using sound and movement (page 75) can also help you tune in to the tree's rhythms. People usually first pick up the rhythms with which they feel some affinity and which are therefore more accessible. To go further, repeat the exercises listening for different rhythms. This brings you closer to discovering the tree and to discovering more of yourself.

CASE STUDY

"As soon as I sat back against this pine tree and calmed down, I was gripped by a strong feeling, like a breath that rose up through my spine, from the sacrum to the back of my neck. Now and again this very direct movement gave way to another kind of breathing, a double movement much less full, with a current going up on the left and coming down on the right, then the opposite. It seemed to be showing me the difference between the oneness of life and the duality of my consciousness."

Guy, workshop participant

EXERCISE 21:
FEELING THE ENERGY FIELD OF A TREE

These steps will enable you to sense the tree's energy field and feel its quality.

❶ PREPARATION

Choose a tree that you feel drawn to spontaneously. Hug the tree, putting your arms around its trunk, and notice what sensations this gives you in your body. Then put your hands flat on the trunk, either at shoulder height or letting your arms hang naturally.

❷ PERCEIVING THE FIELD

With eyes closed and keeping your awareness in the palms of your hands, move back slowly from the tree, lifting your hands off. Notice the sensations in your palms - you may feel tingling, vibration, or something else. Holding your attention in your palms, keep moving slowly backward until the sensation fades. This indicates the outer edge of the field.

❸ FEELING THE LAYERS

Come back to the tree and repeat stage 1. As you move away you will feel a change in the sensation in your hands, which may become more intense or different in quality. This marks a zone of transition between the layers. Go over the sensations in each layer, until you can recognize the zones.

❹ FEELING THE EFFECTS

Position yourself in front of one of the transition zones, with your hands in contact with it, and observe the reactions in your body. Then stand with your whole body in this zone and notice what else happens.

❺ INTEGRATION

Sit against the tree or lie beside it if the ground is comfortable, and pay attention to what you feel and what is coming up - it may be thoughts, images, memories, or new physical sensations.

The more you do this exercise, the more you will discover the secrets of the energy field.

Exercises 21 and 22 will help you to become sensitive to the different layers of the tree's energy field. As you explore them you will become more conscious of your own energy bodies.

EXERCISE 22: *TUNING IN TO YOUR OWN ENERGIES IN THE PRESENCE OF A TREE*

The seven phases of this exercise correspond to the seven levels of consciousness, and if you look closely you will see the analogy with the seven attitudes to the tree we looked at earlier (pages 34-5).

❶ CHOOSE A TREE
See Exercises 10 and 11 on pages 64-5.

❷ FIND A GOOD POSITION
See how you position yourself, sitting or standing, facing the tree, or with your back against it. Does one part of the tree seem welcoming? This is a first step in relating consciously to the tree.

❸ WAIT AND SEE - BUT NOTHING HAPPENS, HOW DISCONCERTING!
This feeling is an indispensable part of every process of change. Feelings and doubts rush in to fill the void: "What am I doing here? Why don't I feel anything?" The mind wanders, old memories pop up from nowhere, the imagination leaps ahead into the future. This is the time to let go of expectations. Just wait.

❹ PAY ATTENTION TO THE SENSATIONS IN YOUR BODY
The only way to unscramble the chaos is to come back into the present. To do this, notice the different sensations your body feels. At first the physical ones are the most obvious, maybe the discomfort, but gradually other more subtle feelings come through.

❺ CONTACT IS MADE
Eventually you begin to feel in contact with the tree, and unexpected and surprising feelings emerge.

❻ RELISH THE SENSATIONS
Explore and enjoy the sensations that come to you. The mind will still be pouncing on them to analyze and explain and label what is happening, but if you can persuade it to stay on the sidelines as an observer then your feeling self will stay available for the actual experience.

❼ YOU AND THE TREE MEET, THE EXCHANGE HAPPENS
At this stage the experience oftens attains the mystical. You feel at peace, at one with the tree, and with nature. Everyone whom I have seen experience this comes back with tears of joy, quite unable to put into words what has happened. The experience itself may last only a few moments, but it will stay with you for the rest of your life.

Don't expect that each phase of the experience will last the same length of time, or even that you will go through all the stages on one occasion. One day you will get stuck at stage 2 because you can't find a position that feels good, another day the problem will be the next stage because your mind can't stop spinning. But the outline above acts as a guide to where you are on the ascending curve of awareness; and one day you will feel pulled irresistibly upward toward the transcendent.

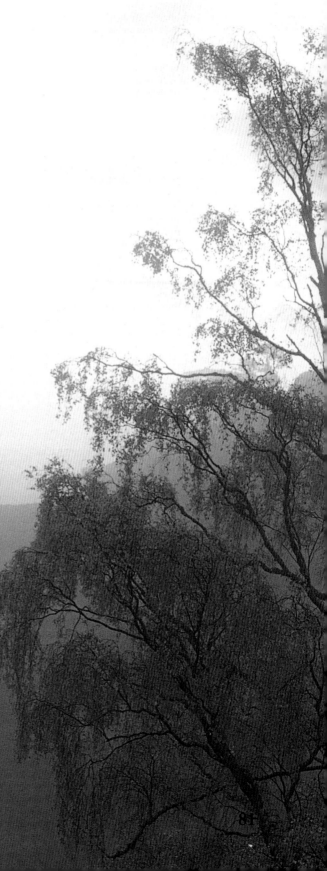

E X E R C I S E 2 3 : *ENCOUNTERING
A TREE WITH YOUR ENERGY BODIES*
Every contact between living beings
brings about an exchange between their
respective energy fields. We are not
usually aware of the process, but in this
exercise you can explore it by sensing
what happens as you approach a tree.

❶ Stand about ten metres (thirty-three
feet) away from a tree, blindfold yourself and walk slowly toward it. Don't
try to memorize where it is, but keep
your sense of direction and let yourself
operate in a different mode, staying
sensitive to all that is going on, in your
body and around you.

❷ When you have done this a few
times you can extend it by going to a
place with many trees and walking
blindfold among them, becoming
aware of their presence.
Take someone with you as a partner, as
in the "guardian angel" exercise (see
page 69), and get them to tell you afterward how close you came to the trees.
Even while blindfolded, people often go
straight for one tree and avoid another,
so ask your partner to tell you which
ones you came close to and which you
stayed away from. If you have time, go
back to a few of them and, as you
begin to sense their different qualities,
ask yourself why you avoided some and
went to meet certain others.

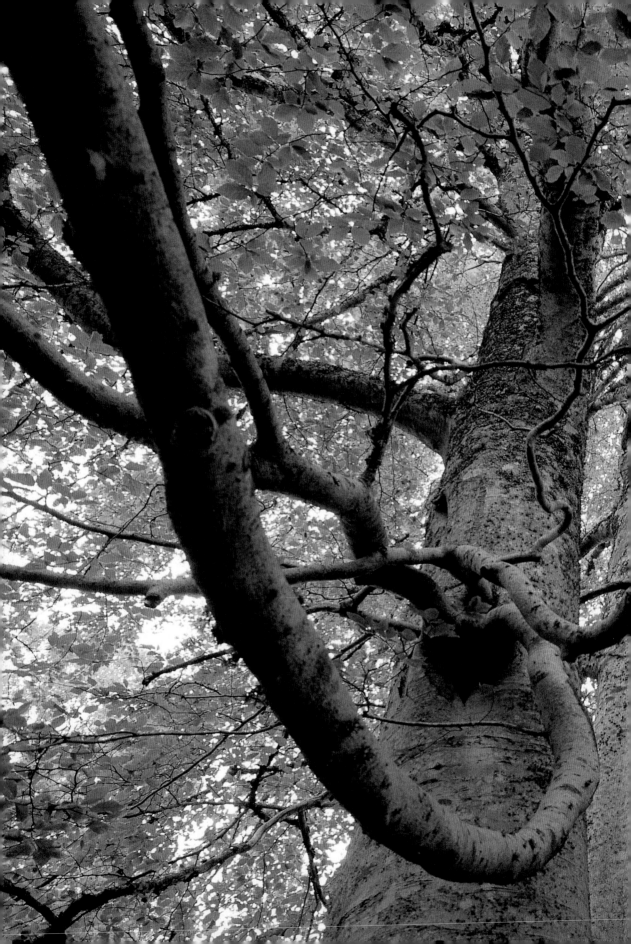

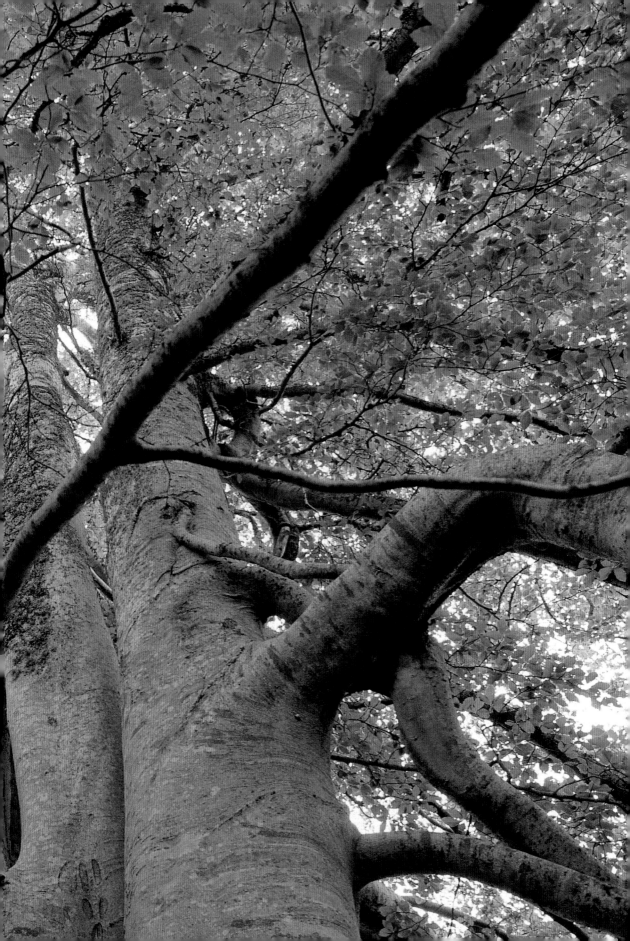

Qualities of trees

Each species of tree has its own distinctive shape and way of producing its flowers, fruits, and seeds, so that it can adapt to the conditions in which it grows. If you observe these characteristics closely you begin to see that each type of tree expresses a certain quality in its habits and in its way of being.

The tree takes its particular form in order to embody its inherent quality. In other words, its physical body conveys specific information and is an expression of the tree's true nature.

Discovering the true qualities of different trees is a fascinating adventure. This exercise (left) give you some practice, and more detailed techniques are presented in Chapter 5.

We have seen that when we enter a tree's energy field our own energy field reacts and adapts to that of the tree. The information a tree embodies is not something that you have to take away from the tree, it is something you can acquire by attuning yourself to it. As when you read a newspaper, the information is still all there when you have taken from it what you want to know. However, some items will interest you and others won't; you will "tune in" to the things that concern you, which stir up feelings, give pause for thought, bring back memories. This process of "tuning in" is called resonance.

As you become more sensitive to the presence of a tree, you will probably find yourself tuning in to its predominant quality, which will in turn make you aware of this quality in yourself. If for instance I stand near a fir tree, which embodies a quality of fluidity, I will gradually sense this fluidity in my

EXERCISE 24: *A FIRST GLIMPSE OF THE QUALITIES OF A TREE*
To get an idea of the quality of a particular tree, start by looking at it as a whole.

❶ Choose a tree that appeals to you and look first at its overall shape. Some words will spring to mind to describe it: majesty, power, strength, gentleness - the first clues to its inherent quality.

❷ Then look more closely at the leaves and see what words come to you. Do these convey the same idea as the first? Take a good look at each part of the tree in turn, at the flowers or fruit if they are present. Look also at the way the tree fits into its surroundings.

❸ Ask yourself the following questions:
What kind of inner attitude does this tree inspire in me?
Confidence, fear, calm, humour, ...
If this tree were a person what would I like to do with him?
What would I like to ask her?
From your answers to these questions and your observations of the tree, one predominant quality should emerge.

own system. The next stage is to notice how I
react to this movement. I may let it happen and
feel better first in my body, freeing my breathing
and releasing tight muscles, then gradually letting
go emotional tensions and some of the limits in my
mind. Or maybe I will refuse this "invitation",
becoming more resistant and more tense, in oppo-
sition to the qualities of the tree. This may be an
instinctive reaction below the level of my awareness, but sooner or later I will become conscious of
it. Whether this takes a few seconds or a few years,
it will in the end bring greater freedom.

Each meeting is unique

When you make a true exchange with a tree, you
will have an experience of an intensity that will
stay with you for the rest of your days. However a
few days later, in the same situation with the same
tree, what happens may be just as intense but quite
different. If you compare notes about it with other
people you will find a third angle. So instinctively
the mind starts to decide who is "right", and that is
an open door to criticism and intolerance.

This sort of thinking is narrow and divisive.
Learning to consider and respect how others
experience reality enriches our own experience,
and makes us more open and curious about people.
The richness of the many faceted world we share is
not a matter of being "right", but of discovering as
many facets as possible.

To see why what you experience is not the
same as for other people, or why it doesn't repeat
itself, remember that the tree has its own energy
field, and that a person approaching the tree goes
through an unconscious process of responding and
adapting to it. Imagine, for comparison, walking in
a town on a dark evening and seeing someone
coming toward you. Probably you feel a stab of
fear, then you try to calm yourself by thinking,
well they're not necessarily going to mug me. You
relax for a moment, then the fear comes back. Just

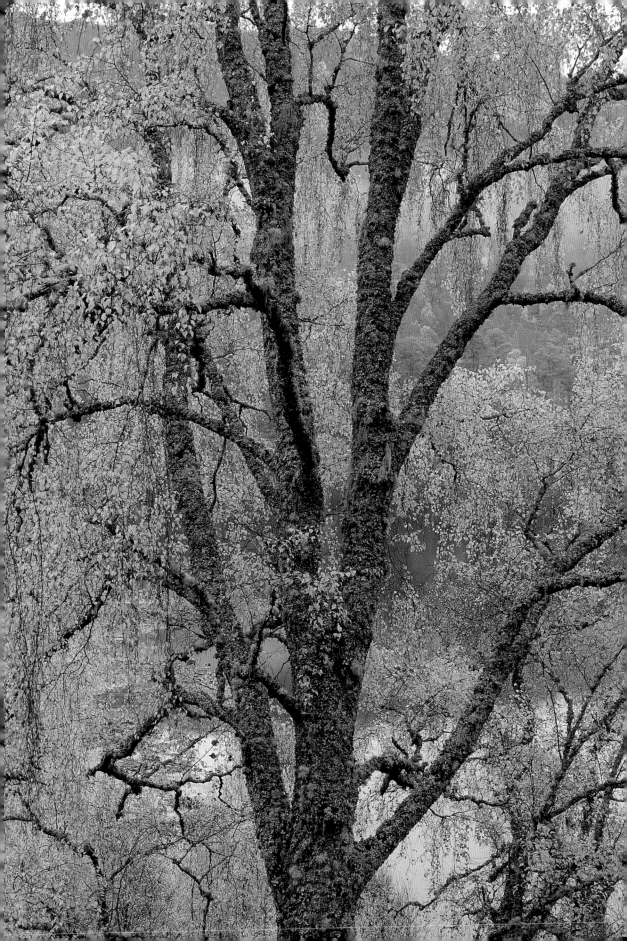

before you pass each other you waver between fear and trust, between doubt and confidence, between being relaxed and being aggressive. Somehow this chaos of feelings resolves as you pass by the other person, who has probably been through the same feelings as yourself. On one evening your fear is uppermost, on others your confidence.

When you enter the energy field of a tree the same sort of dialogue is going on, but out of the hearing of your conscious mind. The reality of the moment is created by the meeting of the two energy fields, tree and person. The energy field of each human being is perpetually shifting, changing quickly in some aspects and more slowly in others. It is only because some attitudes evolve very slowly that we assume there is something permanent about our inner world. Thus to each encounter with the tree we bring some different version of ourselves according to the state we are in at the time, and so no two meetings will be the same.

Through the exercises in this chapter you will have discovered that a tree has an energy field and a specific form which conveys its predominant quality. Some aspects of this quality we can grasp with our senses, but there are other more subtle aspects that we can discover only by tuning in to the inner rhythms of the tree and by making available our own inner rhythms of breathing, sound, and movement. In the next chapter we will focus on the qualities of nine species of trees, from which I have prepared energized oils that embody the characteristic quality of each tree, and which make these qualities accessible as a support on the journey of life.

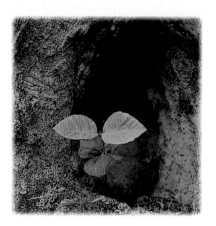

Chapter 4

The healing energies

During the months we spent living in the forest, my wife and I noticed that our aches and pains often disappeared after only a few minutes sitting against a tree trunk. There was no doubt that there was a connection between feeling better physically and the tree's presence, and although it was not always as dramatic as the relief of pain, we noticed how our bodies felt different when we were close to certain trees. The trees' effect was not limited only to physical sensations but also influenced our state of being - some made us feel calm, some more excited, while others imparted feelings of security or of joy.

Through our observations over a long period we were eventually able to select nine trees whose individual qualities are vital to health and wellbeing. By working with their energies you can strengthen and enrich your daily life, freeing blocks in your energy bodies, and becoming more in touch with your higher self. You can also increase your self-esteem and self-confidence, which will empower you to become more open, and to let go of the weight of the past.

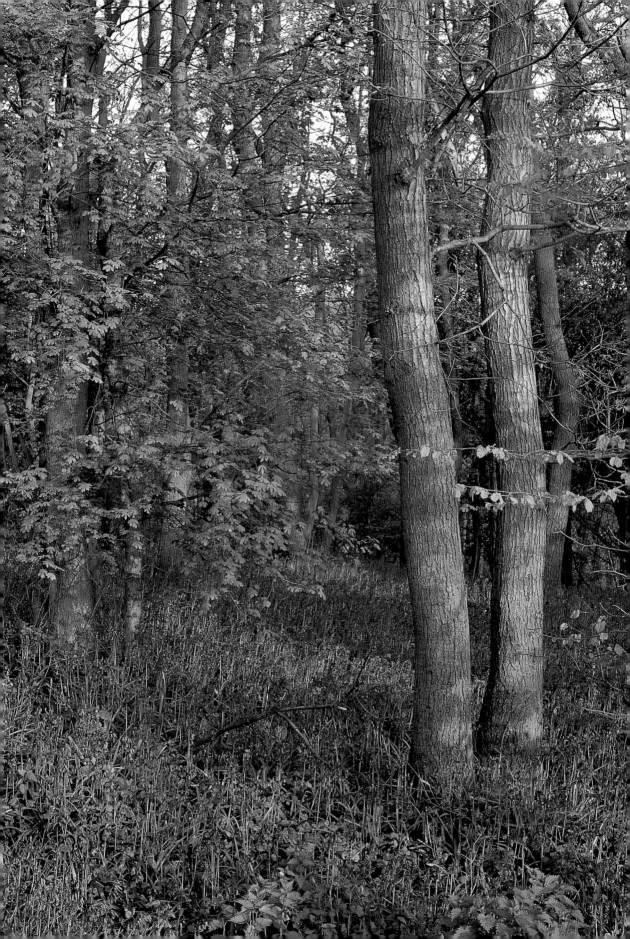

In Chapter 3 we saw how each tree species has an individual quality, shared by all trees in the species, which arouses certain types of sensation within us, for example calm, confidence, or fluidity. These qualities can be perceived in the physical features of the tree, such as the shape of the trunk, its bark, its leaves, and its habitat and role in the ecosystem. In each encounter with a tree your energy field responds to that of the tree, reacting and adapting to it. By attuning to the inner rhythms and energy field of the tree you can absorb the information that it carries - the imprint of its special quality - awakening that quality within yourself.

The qualities of some trees are not particularly relevant to the human experience, but others are vital to our health and wellbeing. In the process of identifying those most beneficial to us, my wife and I made many observations and shared our experiences with others. From this a consistent picture of the qualities emerged. The birch has the gift of gentleness. The beech is never encroached on by undergrowth or parasites: its self-assurance keeps at bay any possible invaders. The hawthorn adapts itself to its situation and grows even with other trees close by, holding its own space without being suffocated or taking what the others need. The fir, a tall tree with a straight trunk, manifests fluidity, while the wild rose embodies openness; pine has a special connection with the light. We chose also the box, which looks more or less the same throughout its annual cycle; the walnut which grows on its own rather than in a wood, and has its own distinctive rhythms; and the broom which comes to life in an explosion of sun-yellow flowers.

The energies of the nine trees presented here offer valuable support at each stage of dealing with an illness or crisis (see Chapter 2). The techniques and exercises for working with these tree energies at the different stages of the process are explained in Chapter 5.

Energized tree oils

Once we had identified the nine trees with the most beneficial qualities we began to explore ways of transferring these precious qualities into some other medium, so that they could be more easily accessible. We decided to use oil, which has a complex structure capable both of absorbing a range of different energies and holding them for a considerable period of time.

Eventually we developed our method for transferring the tree energies into the oil. For each of the nine trees we prepare a mother tincture by soaking parts of the tree in an oil and water emulsion. Nothing is cut or removed from the tree, so it is not harmed at all. The mother tinctures for each species are prepared at times auspicious for the individual trees, and the salinity of the oil and water mixture used is adjusted to match as closely as possible the energy of the tree.

The mother tinctures are incorporated into an organic vegetable base oil, which is solarized (allowed to absorb energy from the sun) in suitable weather conditions. During this process the energy structure of the base oils adapts to the energy pattern of the tincture. Sometimes after a few hours a viscous plasma appears in formations which are different for each oil (see page 93), or there are subtle changes in the colour: the nine oils range from pale yellow through to dark gold. The oils are complex energy structures which are linked with the energy field of the tree species. No logical explanation has been found for these phenomena, which perhaps indicates that there is still much more to learn from them; the behaviour of the oils hints at a wider reality.

Using the oils

We have seen how in a meeting with a tree our energy fields react and adapt to the tree's energy field and attune to its qualities. The energized tree oils work in the same way: the human energy field

91

reacts to the energy patterns of the oil, by adapting and attuning to it. In our conventional system we have a notion of an average requirement of vitamins, minerals, trace elements, etc, and we can work out a dose accordingly to compensate for what we lack. But this approach does not work with an energized oil - we can't prescribe 10mg of gentleness or 150cc of autonomy. Whichever quality you may feel you need at a given time is hidden away inside you somewhere in your higher self, but all too often the ego stops it from coming through. Treatment with the oil awakens the respective quality within you.

The energized tree oils can be taken orally, or used in a bath or for massage, but they are usually applied directly on a part of the body. Whenever you feel a physical pain it is the outcome of something happening in your energy field, so there is always a link beween the problem in the energy body and the place where you feel the physical symptoms. Thus by applying the oil where it hurts, you target the problem on an energetic level. At the same time the problem or blockage in the energy field sets up a vibrational pattern that is echoed in the chakras according to their sphere of influence (see page 44). By applying the oil to a specific chakra you can target fairly accurately a particular aspect of a problem.

The following pages present illustrated profiles of the nine trees and their qualities, as well as the particular benefits of working with the energy of each tree. You can access and work with these energies through the exercises in Chapters 3 and 5, or by using the energized tree oils. The effects of the oil on each chakra are also listed for each tree. For details of how to purchase the oils, see page 160.

A viscous plasma (see right) may appear in the mixture of the mother tincture and the base oil during solarization (see page 91).

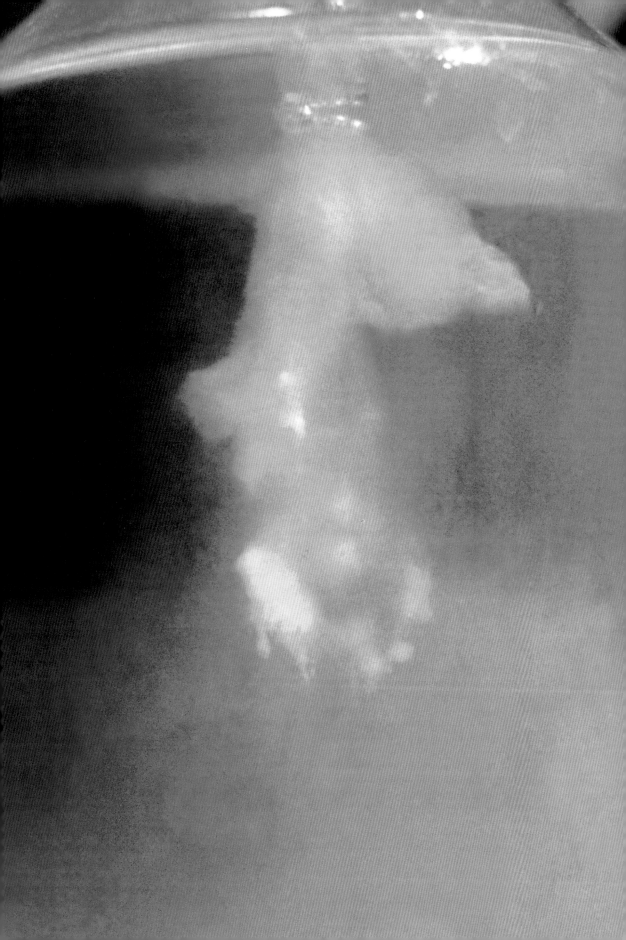

Birch

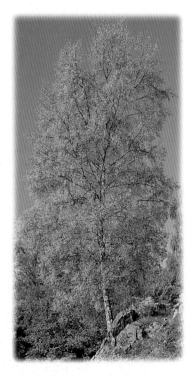

QUALITIES:
GENTLENESS
RECONCILIATION

There are around 40 species of birch (*Betula)* which can be most easily recognized by their smooth white bark and light airy foliage. There is a delicacy in the way the birch's slender branches combine to create its overall shape, and its finely shaped leaves flutter elegantly in the slightest breeze, to be replaced in winter by the catkin-like fruits. The weeping birch, *Betula pendula*, grows in light sandy soil, and other birch species will survive where the soil is poor and thin. In all stages of its growth it keeps a harmony of proportion.

In temperate climes the birch is the first tree to grow back spontaneously after a natural disaster such as an earthquake or volcanic eruption, and even after a nuclear accident. All its features reveal a quality of gentleness and sweetness, but there is nothing feeble about it; under the delicate peeling bark is a hard and sturdy wood.

To sit under a birch is to enter an atmosphere of gentle peace, a reminder that life is not all struggle but can be harmonious and sweet. It is the place to let go of burdens and accept the gifts that life is offering.

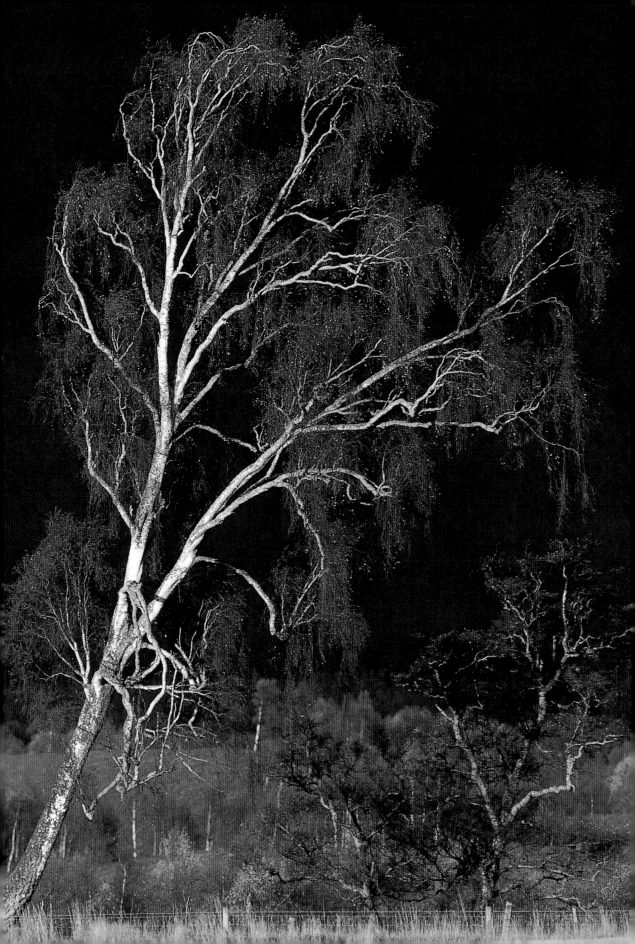

THE ENERGIES OF BIRCH

The birch has the quality of gentleness, which can be used to treat any shock:

● physical shock such as an injury, burn, or severe pain.

● emotional shock ranging from minor problems such as hearing unexpected news, to serious shock such as sudden separation or bereavement.

Birch also has the energy of reconciliation. By helping us become more calm it creates space for peace in our relationship with ourselves and with others.

MAIN MESSAGE:
ACCEPTING AND BECOMING RECONCILED WITH ONESELF GAINING SELF-ESTEEM

RELIEVING TENSION

Pain in the shoulders, jaw, or stomach is often due to tension, since the energy of our life struggle is commonly focused in these areas. The gentleness of birch can help relieve such aches and pains caused by stress.

RECONCILING THE MASCULINE AND FEMININE

In daily life we tend to use mostly our masculine energies of will, ignoring our more gentle feminine energies. The birch helps us to reconcile these two aspects of ourselves and reconnect the link between them, enabling us to function more creatively.

RESOLVING ESCALATING EMOTIONS

Emotions such as anguish, fear, or anger can overwhelm us. We may react to them with guilt, or more anguish and anger, so our feelings escalate, getting more out of hand. The energy of birch helps us to make peace with ourselves, just as we are.

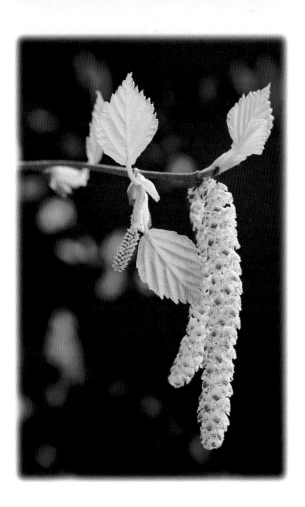

MAKING PEACE WITH THE CRADLE OF LIFE

Gynaecological problems in women may result from the emotional wounds that underlie past experiences, such as abortion, miscarriage, painful periods, etc. The birch helps us to acknowledge such problems and face them with a new attitude.

COPING WITH CHANGE

Surgery or an accident can make a permanent change to the body. The birch can help reconcile us to such changes.

EFFECT ON THE CHAKRAS

BROW
more gentleness in thinking about the problem

THROAT
expressing yourself more calmly

HEART
healing wounds; feeling goodwill toward yourself and others

SOLAR PLEXUS
softening the effect of feelings

HARA
being at peace with yourself

RISING ABOVE THE EGO

Birch energies can help in the effort to tame the ego (learning how it operates so we are no longer its victim) making more room for the higher self to function.

97

Beech

The beech (*Fagus*) is one of the most imposing deciduous trees: its straight trunk rises like a column, reaching heights of up to 45 metres (150 feet). Beech trees have a majestic strength and a serene stability. Their roots spread wide but are not deep, as if the tree hardly needs more than its own self-assurance to keep it upright. The beech can also grow among trees of other species and hold its own in their company. It grows with great vigour and is extremely hardy.

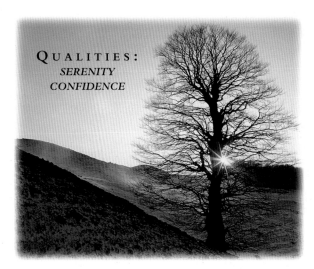

QUALITIES:
*SERENITY
CONFIDENCE*

The beech has the capacity to repel invaders: in a beech wood there is hardly any under-growth, and beech trees are rarely encroached upon by ivy or mistletoe. Another example of this capacity is the antiseptic properties of creosote, a tar extracted from beech wood. In some parts of France the beech is believed to have natural protection from lightning strikes. Further evidence of the beech's quality of resistance is in its wood, which is dense and difficult to work and resists being bent into any shape other than its own.

The beech's strength comes from its inner force and self-assurance and is maintained without struggle. We need to be strong like the beech: to get in touch with the source of inner strength which resolves conflict by radiating calm and assurance.

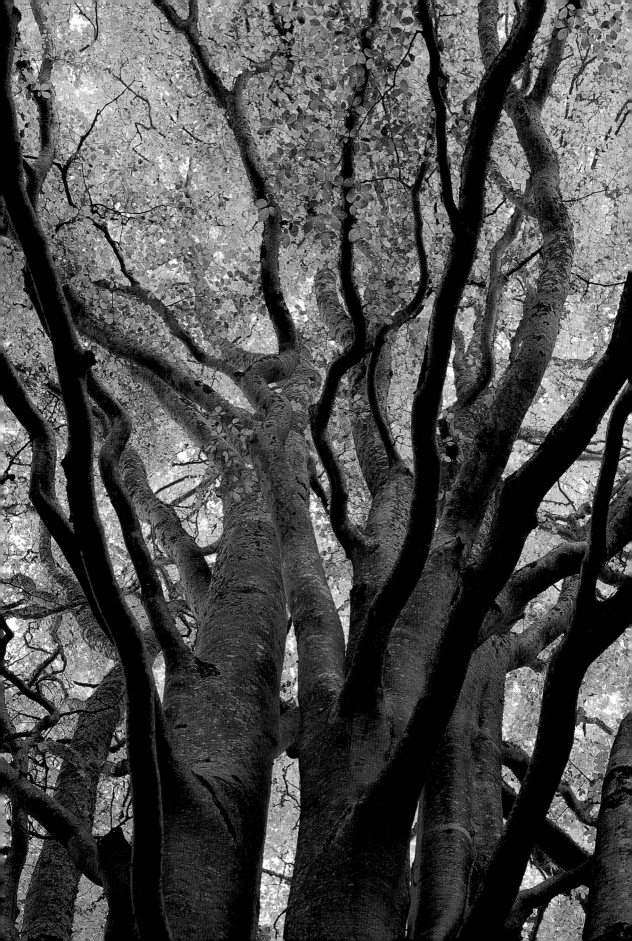

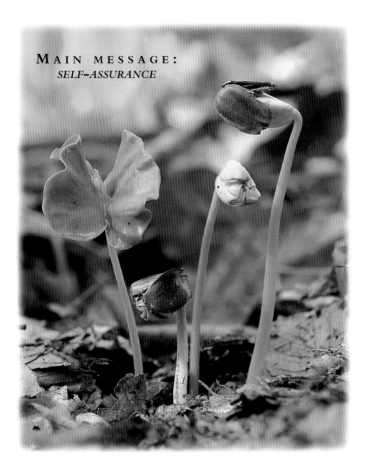

MAIN MESSAGE:
SELF-ASSURANCE

THE ENERGIES OF BEECH

Our daily life is haunted by many fears: of illness, of unemployment, of dying, for our loved ones, our social status, of "doing the wrong thing". We are caught in a vicious circle, where the insecurity we feel creates more fears, which have an effect on our physical and mental health.

Beech's quality of self-assurance awakens in us a sense of serenity, freeing us from our fears and making more space to contact our other qualities.

EFFECT ON THE CHAKRAS

BROW
thinking surely and serenely

THROAT
feeling confident to express yourself

HEART
feeling confident and ready to love

SOLAR PLEXUS
not being swayed by emotions

HARA
contacting your strength and faith in life

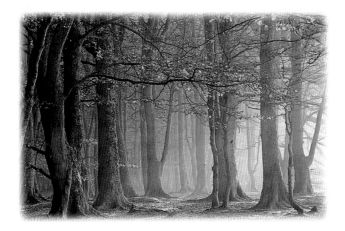

FINDING SELF-CONFIDENCE

Lack of self-confidence makes us doubt not only ourselves and our own capacities, but also others' sincerity or judgement - our lack of faith in them mirrors our own self-doubt. The energy of beech helps our confidence to return, calming the mind enough to make a decision or form an opinion. It is also a valuable support in finding the self-confidence needed to take appropriate action.

TREATING THE PHYSIOLOGICAL EFFECTS OF FEAR

Intestinal problems frequently result from an unconscious inner insecurity caused either by our own thoughts or by contact with other people. The beech encourages an inner change of attitude, so that the body no longer receives the doses of fear that upset it, and can respond more harmoniously. Sore swollen throats often result from energy blocks caused by fear and lack of self-confidence, so can be treated using beech.

OVERCOMING TIMIDITY

Timidity blocks us from being our true selves. Beech helps us to see ourselves more positively and to be more confident.

STRENGTHENING WEAKNESS

Weakness in any part of the body can arise from a sense of vulnerability due to fear. In particular, Chinese medicine recognizes fear as the emotion connected with the kidney. All symptoms of weakness can be treated with the beech.

Fir

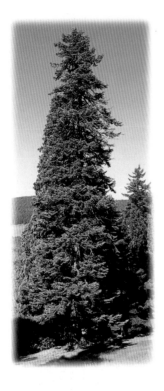

The family of firs (*Abies*) embraces some fifty species, all of which grow symmetrically about a single straight trunk. Fir trees grow quickly, to heights up to 60 metres (200 feet). If the top of the trunk is cut or broken the tree does not grow out to the side or become more bushy, but a new shoot emerges to continue the upward growth. Thus the growth energy appears to act vertically, coming from the crown of the tree, where the cones which carry the seeds cluster. The sap has the same vertical dynamic and is carried from the soil level up to the very tip of the tree.

The trunk is often almost bare of branches, particularly in the darkness of dense forests or plantations, as if the only thing that matters to the pine is for its roots to be anchored in the ground and its crown to be in the light of heaven. In western Europe the spruce, which has similar energies to the fir, is traditionally connected with the birth of a child, when the life of heaven is linked with life on earth. This link between the high and the low, the spiritual and the material, is the special domain of the fir, and is maintained through its fluid energy.

QUALITY:
FLUIDITY

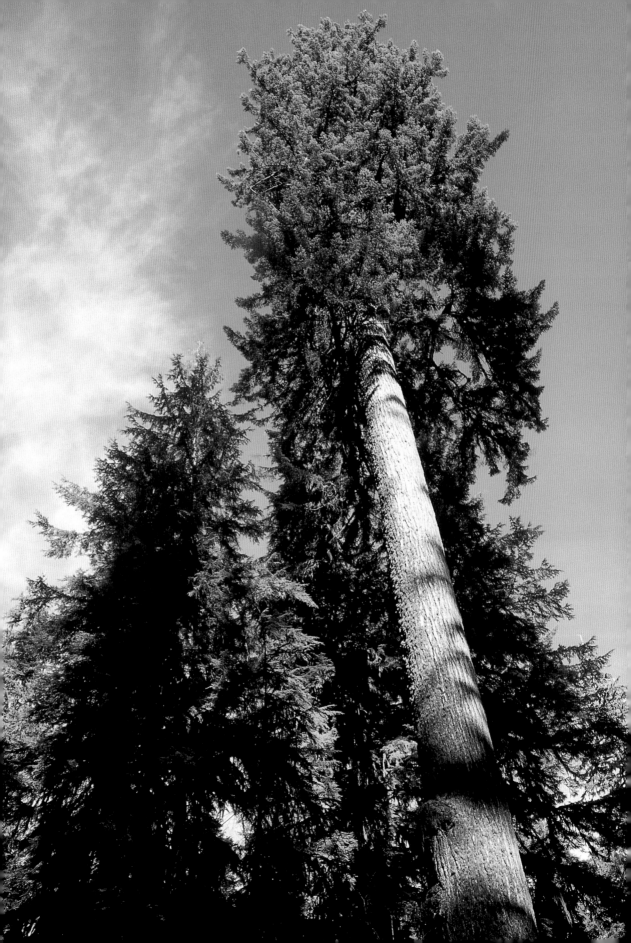

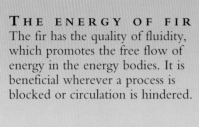

THE ENERGY OF FIR
The fir has the quality of fluidity, which promotes the free flow of energy in the energy bodies. It is beneficial wherever a process is blocked or circulation is hindered.

MAIN MESSAGE:
LETTING GO

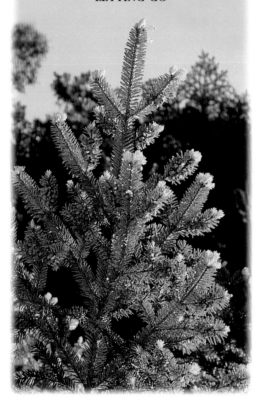

EASING THE BREATHING
Our lungs are more than just empty sacks that we fill with air and then empty. Who we are is revealed in our breathing, which can also indicate the blockages causing our physical symptoms:

● Short, uneven breathing is typical in those who are restless, anxious, or ill at ease.

● Breathing only in the upper part of the chest indicates an over-reliance on mental energy, which can take the place of deeper experience of life.

● Forced breathing indicates a desire to control, which may result from a strong ego and/or a fear of letting go.

The fluid energy of fir works on two levels: to ease the flow of breathing, and to release blockages and smooth the flow in the energy bodies.

EFFECT ON THE CHAKRAS

BROW
accessing the higher
dimensions of yourself

THROAT
expressing your aliveness
with a natural flow

HEART
letting the love in you show
in everything you do

SOLAR PLEXUS
not blocking your feelings

HARA
connecting with the life source

COPING WITH OVERWHELMING EMOTIONS
When our emotions are aroused our breathing alters. In a situation where your feelings overwhelm you, fir supports the breathing and makes these feelings more manageable.

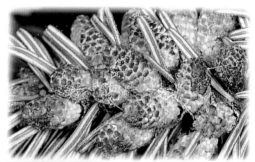

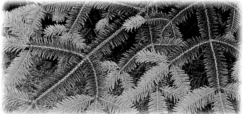

FREEING BLOCKAGES
Problems which appear to result from physical blockages, such as feelings of heaviness in the legs or slow intestinal movements, may actually be caused by blockages in the energy bodies. For a lasting cure these energy blockages must be resolved. The fluidity of fir helps to promote the smooth flow of energy.

105

Pine

The genus *Pinus* includes more than a hundred species. In a mixed forest around dusk you will notice that the pine seems to hold on to the light longer than the other trees. While other trees' foliage is fading into the dark, the pine branches and trunks are still gleaming. The pine is a tree of light and of sunshine: even its bark has the ability to capture the light. The vigorous growth of its shiny needles reminds us that on Earth light is the source of life itself. The pine cones that carry the tree's seeds show the same vitality.

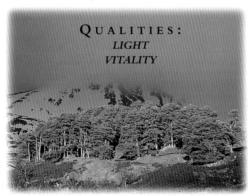

QUALITIES:
LIGHT
VITALITY

The pine bears both male and female flowers on the same tree and so is self-fertile, and in a sense a bearer of life. Attis, the god of fruitfulness and fertility worshipped in ancient times throughout Asia Minor and Greece, was associated with a sacred pine tree which died and came back to life again.

Pine trees are modest in their demands and can live on next to nothing. They will anchor themselves in the most barren soil, even surviving in the minimum of earth on nearly bare rock, as if the light provides for their needs. This reminds us that we too, though anchored on the earth, need the light of heaven for our survival.

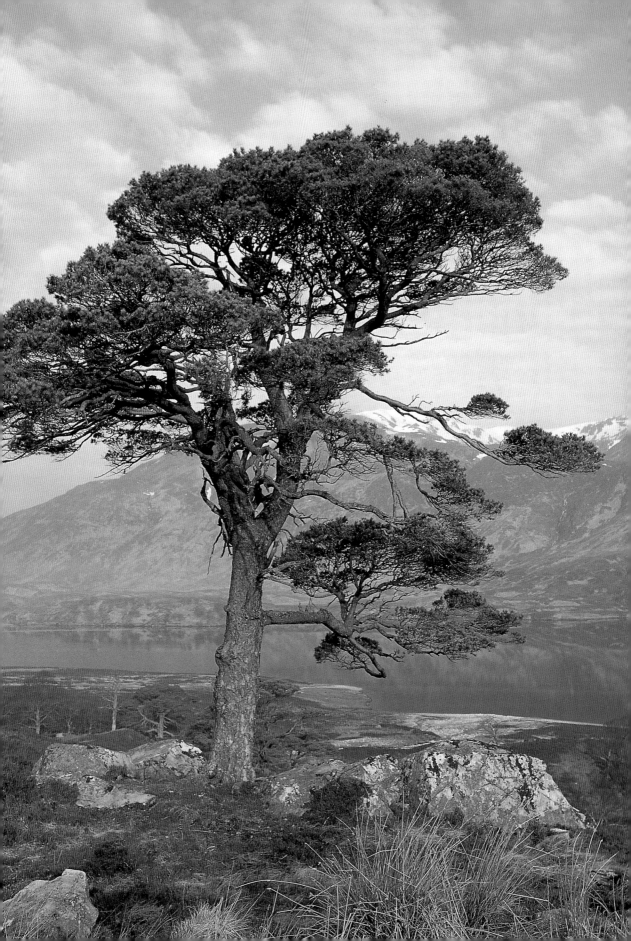

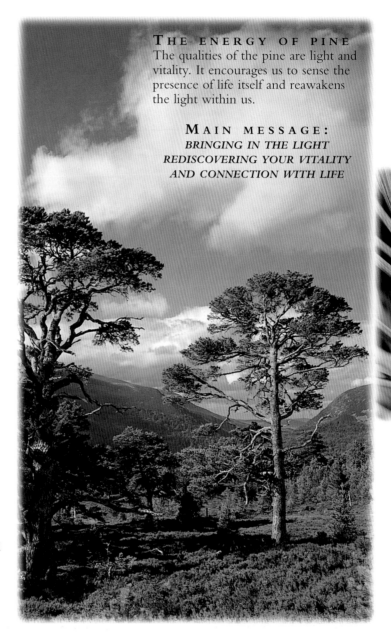

THE ENERGY OF PINE

The qualities of the pine are light and vitality. It encourages us to sense the presence of life itself and reawakens the light within us.

MAIN MESSAGE:

BRINGING IN THE LIGHT
REDISCOVERING YOUR VITALITY
AND CONNECTION WITH LIFE

RELEASING LIMITS

We work within limits that are self-imposed and define and identify with this limited version of ourselves. Our problems can seem enormous because we only see them from our limited perspective, and we may feel lost in the darkness.

Our limits come from our personal history. They should not be ignored or denied - we need to let our inner light grow stronger to free us from them. You can stay on the threshold of a darkened room feeling afraid, or you can enter and open the shutters. As soon as the daylight enters, the frightening shadows disappear.

The pine helps us to see the light in any situation which, from within our limitations, looks dark and desperate.

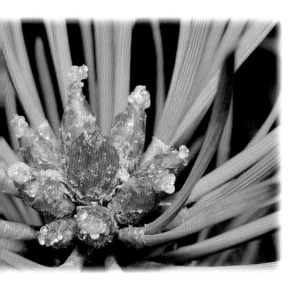

EFFECT ON THE CHAKRAS

BROW
clarifying ideas; seeing more clearly

THROAT
expressing yourself; manifesting
the joy of life

HEART
feeling the joy of being alive

SOLAR PLEXUS
lightening your feelings,
recycling emotional energy

HARA
strengthening vitality by
accessing the life force

CONNECTING WITH LIFE

Nowadays we spend a lot of time in ideas
and inventions, which have nothing to do
with what is truly alive. We get trapped in
the ego's tendency to categorize and label
objects and events and people, but this cuts
us off from their essence - their living part.
Sometimes when a situation seems hopeless
we may feel that we are being carried along
by the force of life which moves on in spite
of us. But in fact we are still being guided
by another level of ourselves. We need to
recognize this and give it space.

The energy of the pine reminds us that we
have a spark of life within us. Though our
limits block and restrict it, the flow of this
life force cannot be stopped.

RENEWING ENERGY

Our disconnection with life, and the limits
that restrict us, affect our energy levels and
may have physiological effects such as:
- fatigue
- weakness
- sluggish organ function
- depression

Pine helps us to rediscover our vitality and
connection with life and maintain this
renewed energy. In awakening our inner
light, it also helps us to avoid depression.

109

Hawthorn

QUALITY:
ALIGNMENT

The hawthorn (*Crataegus*) can often live for several hundred years, growing from the bush form into the stature of a real tree.

In their natural state, trees that grow close together shape themselves in one of two ways: either growing away from each other or fusing into what appears to be a single tree. But the hawthorn has found another way to grow. It is not invasive and neither does it let itself be invaded – it always finds a way to adapt and live its life in its own space. Because of this facility for adaptation, the hawthorn does not have a typical shape: some are round, others take the shape of a fan or an arrow, or some other form. This adaptability has also given rise to around 35 different species of hawthorn, which flourish in a wide range of soils.

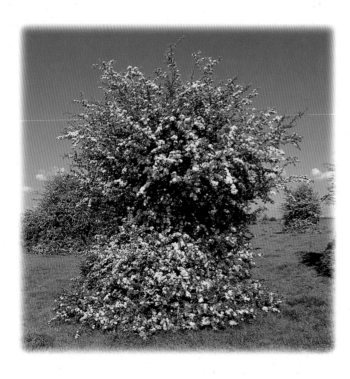

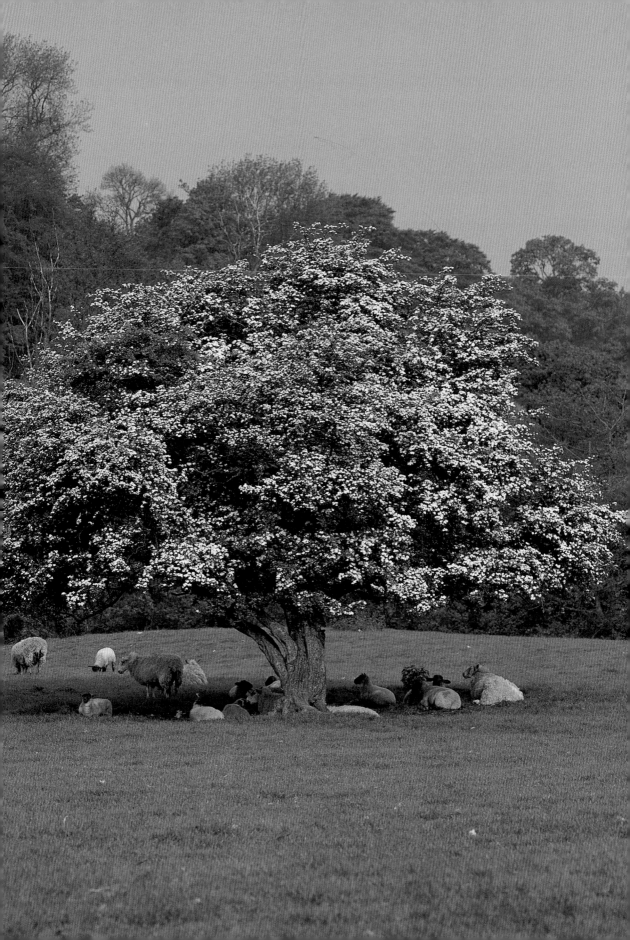

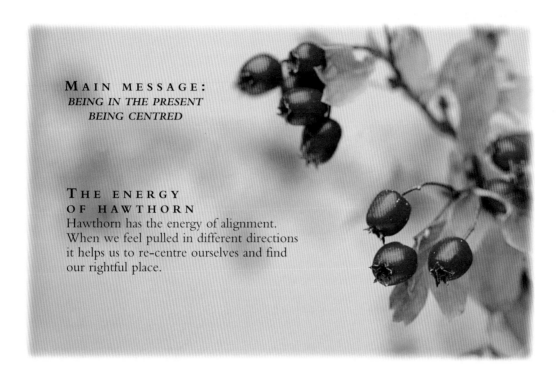

MAIN MESSAGE:
BEING IN THE PRESENT
BEING CENTRED

**THE ENERGY
OF HAWTHORN**
Hawthorn has the energy of alignment.
When we feel pulled in different directions
it helps us to re-centre ourselves and find
our rightful place.

BEING CENTRED IN OURSELVES
The demands of daily life leave us feeling
disoriented, or "not all there". When we
are centred in ourselves, we feel at peace
with what is happening. The energies of
hawthorn help us to centre ourselves.

BEING "AT HOME" IN THE BODY
Many of us have lost touch with our bodies,
through trying to fit ourselves into the
mould dictated by fashion or society. This
cuts us off from an inner awareness of the
body, which is the home of our soul and
so can teach us much about ourselves.
Hawthorn can help us feel at home in the
body, so that by listening to it we can
learn from it.

BEING IN THE PRESENT

So much of the time we live between past memories and the hopes of a distant future. But we need to be in the present if we want to be in touch with reality and all the opportunities it offers us. Hawthorn makes it easier to be there.

EFFECT ON THE CHAKRAS

BROW
concentrating; gathering your thoughts

THROAT
focusing how you express yourself

HEART
loving yourself so you can love others better

SOLAR PLEXUS
not being fragmented by your feelings

HARA
recentring yourself

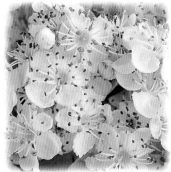

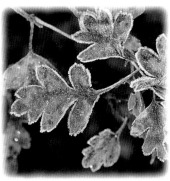

MAKING DECISIONS

If we are cut off from our inner selves we may look to others for advice and solutions to our problems. The aligning energies of hawthorn put us in touch with our inner wisdom so that we can make the choice that is truly best for us.

Wild rose

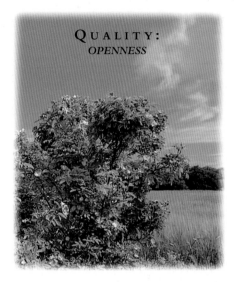

QUALITY:
OPENNESS

Even when it is well established, the wild rose (*Rosa canina*) does not have a distinctive structure of trunk and branches. Its characteristic energy shows itself in its flowering - the vitality of the plant goes into the opening of its flowers.

Many flowering plants blossom when they reach a point of maturity and the flowers may last for several days or even weeks. In contrast the wild rose has a continual succession of blooms. As soon as each flower is completely open, its petals fall. You may admire a spray of wild roses in full flower, but only a few hours later it will already have faded. But after it come dozens and dozens of others which will go on opening throughout the flowering period. Although each flower is over so soon, the flowering period is long, because everything in this plant demonstrates opening that continues without limit or end.

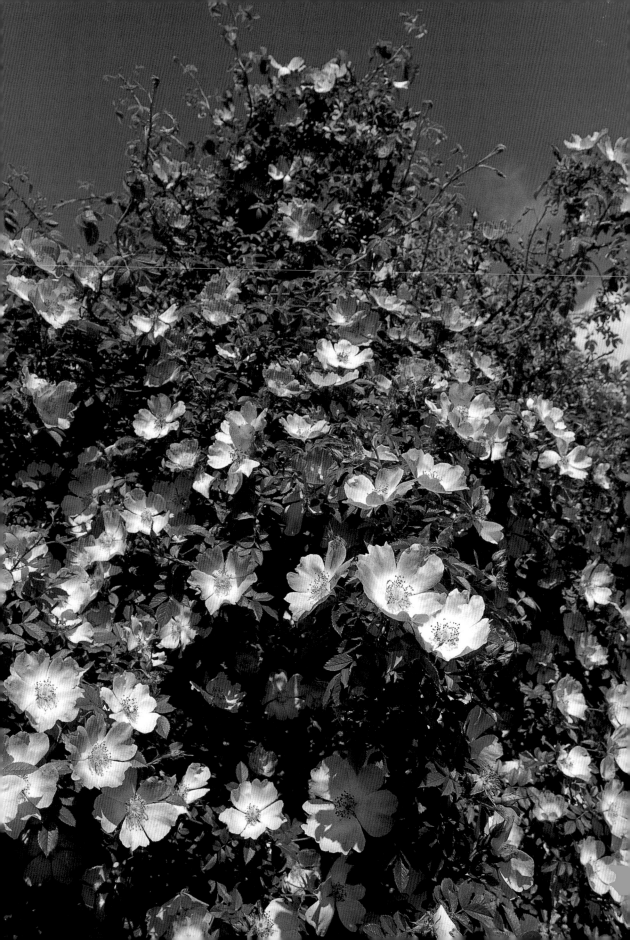

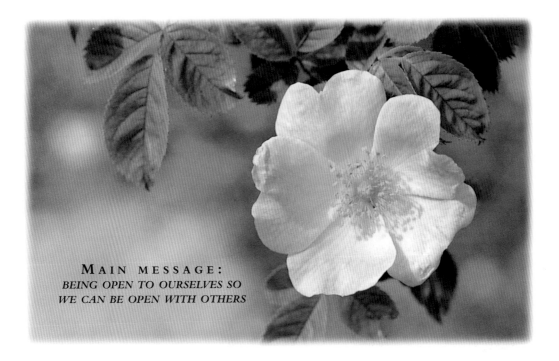

MAIN MESSAGE:
*BEING OPEN TO OURSELVES SO
WE CAN BE OPEN WITH OTHERS*

THE ENERGIES OF WILD ROSE

From our earliest years we become used to being labelled: "You're no good at drawing"; "You're lazy". We begin to believe in these judgements and that it is impossible for us to be any different. Sometimes such labels are convenient because they excuse our failures and explain those aspects of ourselves we do not like.

The problem lies not in the judgement itself but in how we react to it. These beliefs about ourselves create a picture that restricts and limits us. The wild rose's quality of openness helps to free us from these limits.

GROWING THROUGH OUR PROBLEMS

Our tendencies to hide behind our beliefs or avoid reality shape our attitudes to problems that arise. We see them as something external that we must fight against. But a problem or illness is always an invitation to deepen our understanding.

The wild rose helps us to open and gain a different perspective, so that what may seem a serious problem one day is no longer so the next.

EFFECT ON THE CHAKRAS

BROW
releasing your mental limitations

THROAT
developing expression and
openness to others

HEART
showing expansive love

SOLAR PLEXUS
being open to your feelings

HARA
being open to your self

RELEASING OUR TENSIONS

Closedness can show up in the body
in different ways:
- tight mouth and rigid jaw
- frowning
- hunched shoulders
- tightness in the belly or buttocks

All these symptoms reveal deeper
levels of closedness in the self.
Consider when these tensions show
themselves. After which events,
discussions, or thoughts? With
which people?
The wild rose supports and nurtures
this process of growing self-awareness
that can result in a moment of opening, of feeling better, as the aches
and pains disappear.

BEING OPEN WITH OTHERS

According to the stereotype, a closed person is someone
turned in on himself who rarely speaks or smiles, while an
open person is the opposite. But these attitudes are not a
fixed part of the personality. We may be open at certain
moments, with certain people, in certain circumstances,
but closed at others. Wild rose encourages us in self-
expression and being more open in our relationships.

WIDENING OUR VIEW OF REALITY

Our mental energy is often spent on
imagining how things could be, or how
we would like them to be, and we tend to
see each illness or problem as a barrier to
this state of bliss. We may avoid reality by
pinning all our hopes on the future, or by
sinking into regret or disappointment
about the past.
The wild rose helps to bring us closer to
genuine openness, where our view of reality
can grow and create a new inner space.

117

Box

Box (*Buxus*) grows in diverse climates and soils, and in different latitudes. Although it is classed as a sub-Mediterranean shrub it is found throughout central Europe, as well as in Japan. It often grows near monasteries, wayside crosses, standing stones, and in other places of spiritual activity, prompting the theory that for healthy growth box needs a balance of earth and cosmic energies.

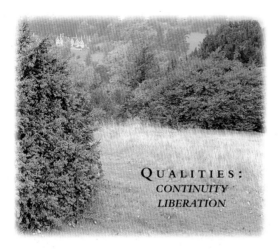

QUALITIES:
CONTINUITY
LIBERATION

Box grows slowly and can live up to six hundred years, and so has become a symbol of longevity. Its foliage is not evergreen, but the tree appears green all year round because it is self-fertile and continually renews itself. Also, the leaves remain green for several months after being cut. Since its flowers and fruits are unobtrusive, box has a constancy of appearance that has led to its becoming the symbol of the perpetual renewal of nature.

Box is used in the Catholic "ceremony of branches" on the Sunday before Easter. The faithful attach a spray of box to a crucifix as a symbol of their faith in the continuity of life. A week later the Resurrection at Easter reminds us that life cannot be destroyed.

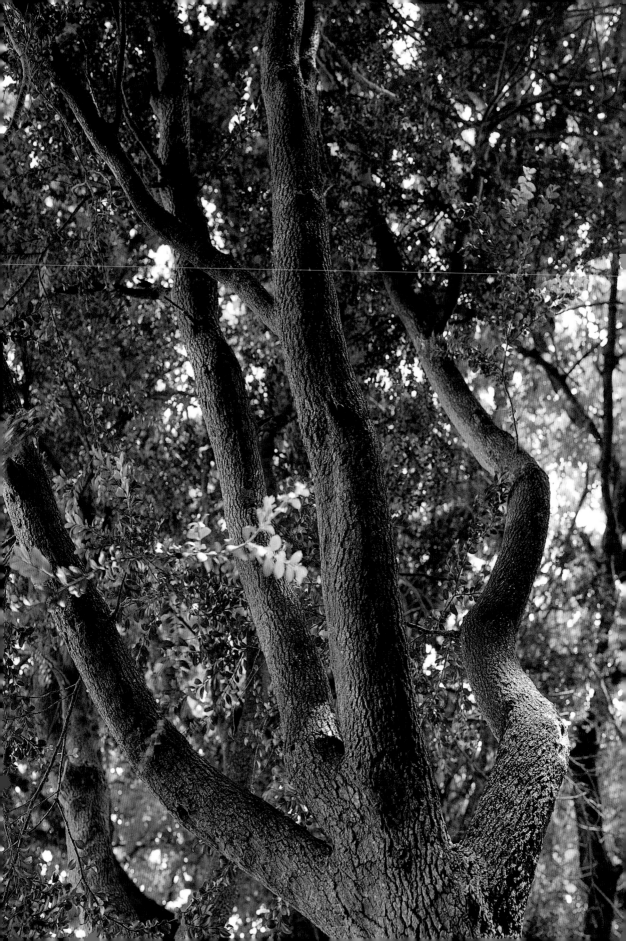

THE ENERGIES OF BOX

Our lack of confidence in the continuity of life means that we tend to accumulate stagnant energy, in fear that life will not provide us with any more. Box has the qualities of continuity and liberation, which help us rise above these doubts and release the blocked energy.

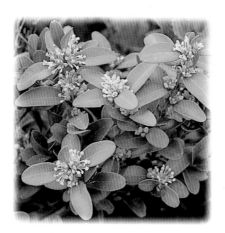

EFFECT ON THE CHAKRAS

BROW
freeing yourself from obsessional thinking

THROAT
expressing what has been blocked

HEART
freeing yourself from the wounds of love

SOLAR PLEXUS
freeing yourself from feelings buried
in deep-seated blockages

HARA
accessing deep-seated blockages

FREEING THE PHYSICAL BODY

Unresolved past experiences often show up in the physical body as chronic illness. Asthma, eczema, ulcers, and intestinal problems may all indicate a blockage in the causal body. Box helps us to become free of the past to clear these blockages.

MAIN MESSAGE:
BECOMING FREE OF THE PAST
RECONNECTING WITH THE
CONTINUITY OF LIFE

FREEING THE EMOTIONAL BODY

It is easy to get stuck with an emotional dynamic that causes certain situations to repeat themselves, for example allowing yourself to be exploited at work. Box can help us take a step toward understanding and freeing ourselves from this dynamic. Phobias and unexplained fears are reactions that are out of proportion to a situation. Box can help us understand these reactions and liberate ourselves from them.

FREEING THE MENTAL BODY

We can become imprisoned by fixed ideas, or blocked by the mistaken ideas we have about ourselves, and these repetitive thought patterns can bring about the same results time and again, such as defeat in work situations, in relationships, problems with money. The energy of box helps to free us from these fixed ideas and patterns.

RELEASING BLOCKAGES IN THE CAUSAL BODY

The memories of our past experiences are held in the causal body. Any "scars" here affect the other energy bodies, and can create difficulties and pain in our mental, emotional, and physical lives. Box helps us to free ourselves from the blockages in the causal body that we carry from the past.

RECONNECTING WITH THE HIGHER SELF

We tend to be cut off from the immortal life force present in us all, hiding behind a screen created by the ego. Box helps us to reconnect with the continuity of life and our higher self.

Walnut

In the natural world the walnut (*Juglans*) does not grow in a wood or in a group, but on its own, in a field or beside a road. It has an independence and autonomy, which reveals itself in its rhythms.

All trees follow the rhythms of the seasons and of day and night, but also have their own subtle rhythms (see page 78). The walnut's individual rhythms have an unusual sequence and emit a strong stimulating energy, which makes it difficult to sleep under a walnut tree.

The complexity of the walnut's branches reflects these different rhythms that it expresses simultaneously. The nut looks like the human brain, the organ which gives the human being the capacity to differentiate from the group and to be autonomous.

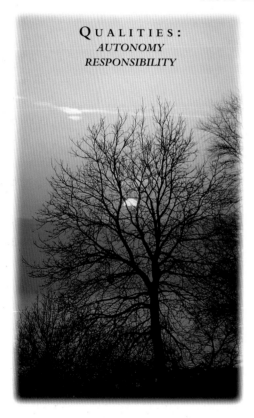

QUALITIES:
AUTONOMY
RESPONSIBILITY

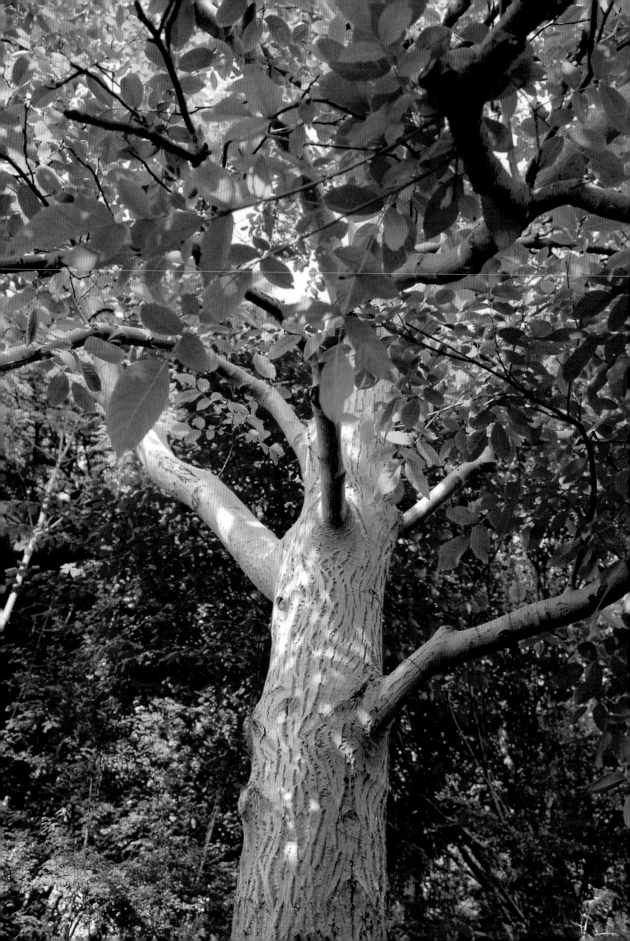

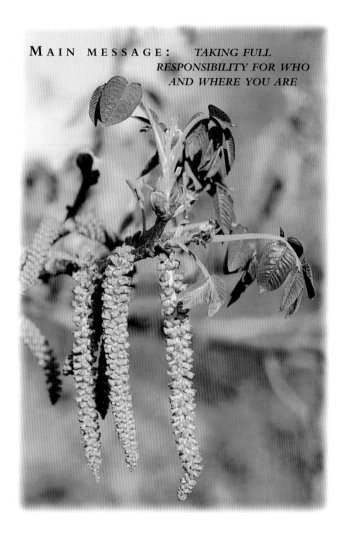

MAIN MESSAGE: *TAKING FULL RESPONSIBILITY FOR WHO AND WHERE YOU ARE*

THE ENERGY OF WALNUT

The walnut encourages us to follow our own rhythms to develop a sense of autonomy and responsibility.

True autonomy comes from within and is reached when we no longer try to avoid facing ourselves. It is seeing ourselves as we really are that creates inner freedom, which allows us to glimpse another reality within us - our higher self. Autonomy creates the space for our higher self to express itself.

124

CHANGING OUR PERSPECTIVE ON WORK

For many of us work is something that has to be endured in order to fulfil our basic needs. The walnut energies help us to see our work in a wider sense, as part of what we are doing in the world, thus giving it a new place in our lives. This may bring up deeper questions of where we are going and why, but the walnut releases the energy to cope with any necessary change.

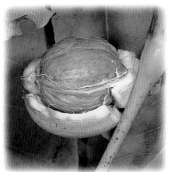

ESCAPING FROM EMOTIONAL PATTERNS

The feelings that upset our relationships with others often follow a pattern that repeats itself again and again. Autonomy means allowing these feelings to appear, facing them, and being able to say at each moment "Just now this is how I am". The walnut facilitates the process of acknowledging our true feelings and thought patterns.

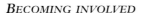

BECOMING INVOLVED

The inner attitude that develops through working with walnut reveals itself in new ways of relating to other people. The changes may not be earth-shattering, but there is a new impetus to be really involved in what we are doing.

EFFECT ON THE CHAKRAS

BROW
learning to distinguish between your illusions and reality

THROAT
having the courage to express what you have chosen

HEART
loving more responsibly

SOLAR PLEXUS
taking charge of your feelings

HARA
revealing who you are; making choices

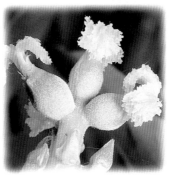

SEEING CLEARLY

The energies of walnut help to bring us back to the real world, and so are helpful when we are indecisive due to an inability to see clearly. A distancing from reality often shows up in the body as irregularities of function in the respiratory or cardiac systems, which will benefit from using walnut energies.

Broom

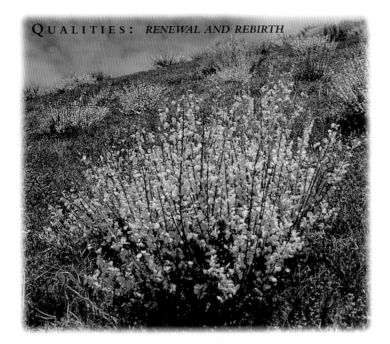

QUALITIES: *RENEWAL AND REBIRTH*

Broom (*Cytisus*) appears in various forms, but all show the same unusual feature. The small, delicate leaves grow on hard angular shoots or stems. Those at the base of the stem each have three lobes and are attached with a stalk, while those at the top of the stem are simple leaves with no stalk. This difference in the form of the leaves between one end of the shoot and the other seems to indicate that the leaves and the stems originally came from two species which through crossing were reborn in the broom.

Thus the qualities of broom are renewal and rebirth, as evidenced by the bright yellow flowers that grow from the previous year's growth. The broom's roots fix nitrogen, feeding and renewing the soil it grows in, and although the broom burns readily in fire, it soon grows back again, being reborn from its ashes like the mythical Phoenix.

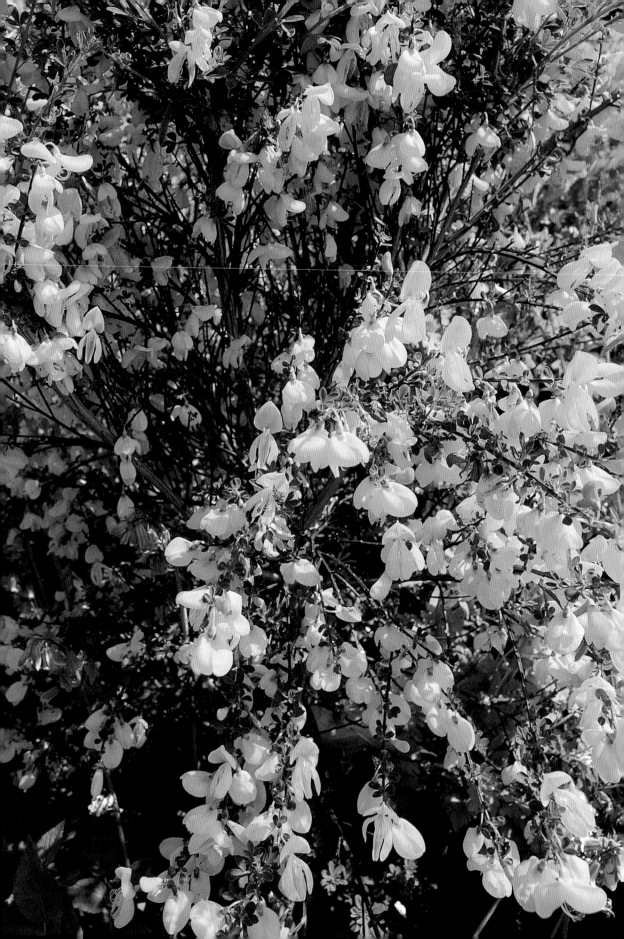

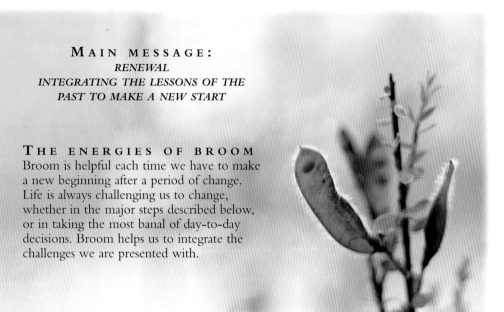

MAIN MESSAGE:
RENEWAL
INTEGRATING THE LESSONS OF THE
PAST TO MAKE A NEW START

THE ENERGIES OF BROOM

Broom is helpful each time we have to make a new beginning after a period of change. Life is always challenging us to change, whether in the major steps described below, or in taking the most banal of day-to-day decisions. Broom helps us to integrate the challenges we are presented with.

BIOLOGICAL CHANGES

The first event of our lives that takes us from one level of energy to another is birth. Puberty is the next, where we suddenly realize that we are different from how we were before. For women, pregnancy and the menopause also involve a similar shift in energy levels. For each of these major life experiences, the aspects that we accept or reject create the patterns that influence how we are for the rest of our lives.

LIFE EVENTS

Between the major biological events, we are faced with many other life situations that invite us to adapt and to transform, for example, weaning, learning to walk, starting school, the first sexual relationship, starting work, marriage, the birth of children. Each is a step that allows us to progress.

RELEASE AFTER CHANGE

After any change at work or in your professional life, the energies of broom make it possible to start anew with all your faculties available.

EFFECT ON THE CHAKRAS

BROW
gaining a new perspective

THROAT
expressing the new energies you feel

HEART
being reborn to life and love

SOLAR PLEXUS
integrating an emotional shock

HARA
allowing new energies to flow in

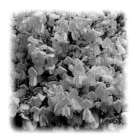

CONVALESCENCE
The release of blocked energy that is signalled by your recovery from a physical illness, or the resolution of a problem, creates a new energy pattern (see page 60). The stage of convalescence is often sacrificed to the need to return to work, or because we want to forget the illness as quickly as possible, but for recovery to be complete it is important to adapt to this new pattern. Broom's quality of renewal and rebirth facilitates the embodiment of the new energetic pattern.

BEREAVEMENT
Broom is a support during the period following the death of someone close, facilitating a release of energy that sets you free, as well as the one who has died.

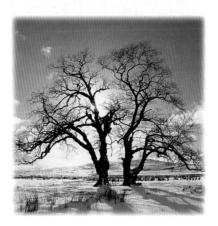

Chapter 5

Healing with tree energies

The quality of a tree reveals itself in many aspects and on many levels; the keys to its discovery are careful observation and a sincere desire to come closer to the truth of the tree. What makes the effort worthwhile is that the qualities present in the tree awaken similar vibrations in ourselves, with far-ranging beneficial effects that enhance our physical, emotional, and mental wellbeing and increase our awareness of our spiritual nature.

The experience of observing and making a deeper contact with a tree can highlight for us how our everyday attitudes affect and limit how we see what is around us. By moving beyond our ordinary thinking patterns we can bring the everyday closer to the life we dream of living. Approaching life in this way means being less obsessed by the circumstances of our problems and more free to look at which of our life tasks we are being asked to work on. This awareness is our first step on the escape route from these limitations and toward enjoying the creativity trapped within them, thus enriching our lives and transforming day-to-day problems.

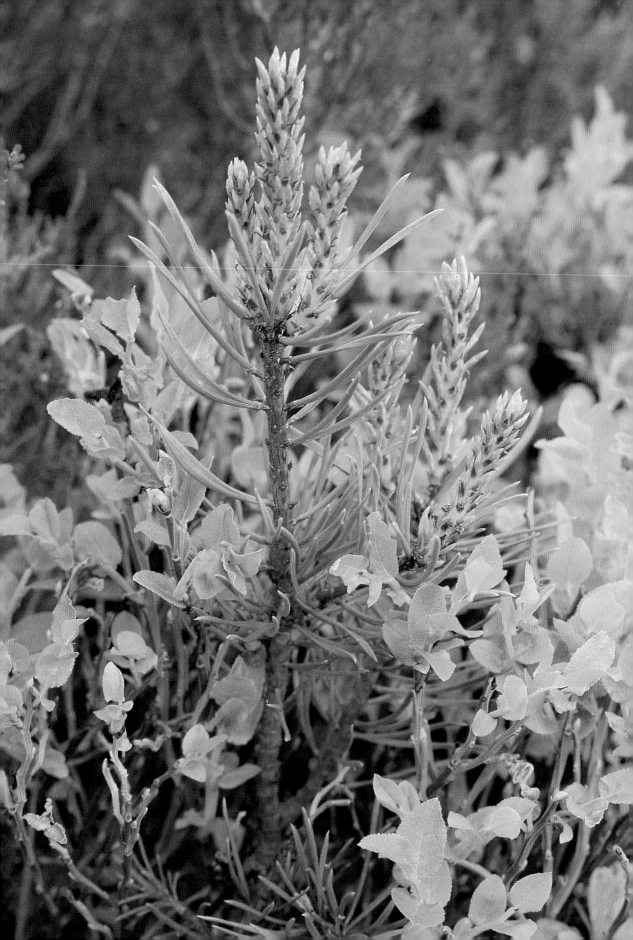

In order to make a deeper contact with trees, you first need to go to the nearest place where a number of trees grow together, such as a patch of woodland or forest. Once you are there, don't waste time regretting your choice and thinking it might have been better to go somewhere else – with this type of attitude you will miss all that the trees have to offer you. The point is not to find a place that is perfect, but to pay attention to what is going on in the place where you are. Focus on discovering what qualities are present in the part of the wood where you are (Exercise 25).

Finding the tree energies you need

To find a tree which can help you with a specific problem, first look at the problem itself, not on the level where it upsets you, but from the perspective of qualities. Ask yourself questions in the present moment. "Now that I'm here and faced with this problem, what qualities do I need right now?" For example, if the problem is "Other people don't make any move toward me" ask yourself: How can I be more open and outgoing to others so they will want to come closer to me? What quality in me is missing that might help this to happen?

Once you have identified a quality that you need, the next stage is to find a tree that holds these qualities. You may have already identified these qualities in a tree you have encountered, using Exercise 26. Another approach is to focus on the quality you are seeking and allow yourself to be guided to a tree with this quality in a walking meditation (Exercise 10, page 64).

You do not need to have a pressing problem uppermost in your mind to benefit from working with tree energies. Once you have discovered both the qualities of the place (Exercise 25) and the qualities of the trees that appeal to you in this place (Exercises 24 and 26), consider what these trees are offering, and in what way this answers your needs of the moment. Ask yourself what else you feel the

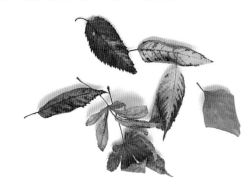

EXERCISE 25: DISCOVERING THE QUALITIES IN A PLACE

Choose a place outdoors that interests you, and seat yourself in it comfortably. Look around you, pay attention to the noises and sounds, to the smells.

What feelings does this place arouse in you?
What do you feel like doing here?
Would you come here to do something in particular? What?
Who would you like to come here with?
What would you do or share?
How would you sum up the quality of this place?

Once you have discovered the qualities of the place, you can see what part the trees play in creating it. Notice which trees appeal to you and observe what it is that you like about them. Exercise 24 (page 84) gives you a first glimpse of the qualities they embody. By observing a tree over a period of time you can make a deeper assessment of its qualities, using Exercise 26.

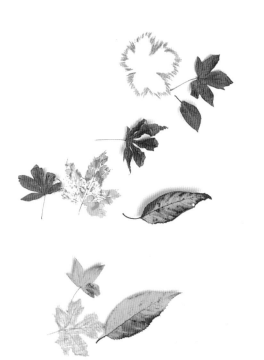

EXERCISE 26: DISCOVERING THE QUALITIES OF A TREE

To gain a deeper insight into the energy qualities of a tree, record your observations over a period of at least one year so that you can observe it in the different seasons.

❶ THE INFORMATION CARRIED BY THE SHAPE OF THE TREE
Observe its silhouette both in winter and in summer. How would you describe it?
Slender, compact, majestic, strong, ...

❷ YOUR REACTIONS TO THE TREE
What response does this tree inspire in you?
Respect, sympathy, a sense of order, strength, letting go, joy, ...

What do you want to do in the presence of this tree?
Relax, reflect, enjoy it, study it, centre yourself, ...

What is most special about this tree?
Which parts of it make the strongest impression?

What is your physical reaction to this tree?
You want to stay, you want to go, you feel drawn toward it, ...

❸ THE INFORMATION GATHERED FROM YOUR SENSES
Use Exercises 12–17 in Chapter 3 to explore the tree in the different seasons: its bark, leaves, sap, flowers, and fruit.
Note the qualities that you observe through each of your five senses. Choose a single word, or as precise a description as possible, to help sharpen your perception.

❹ THE MAIN QUALITY
From all your observations, the main quality of the tree will emerge.

need of, and what qualities you would like to get in touch with. With these answers in mind, make a walking meditation (Exercise 10, page 64) and let yourself be led toward these qualities.

Also notice which trees you are not drawn to: perhaps you find them unappealing or even unpleasant in some way. These may also indicate some of the qualities that would be beneficial to you at this time (Exercise 27).

Focusing on a problem

You can also go into the woods with a specific problem or need in mind: maybe a need for more energy, for clarification, for tenderness, or to find out where you really are. Whatever your need is, the forest can bring you sometimes surprising benefits.

In order to be open to the help in solving your problems that trees can offer, make way for the unexpected. Followed with an open mind, Exercises 28 and 29 can lead you to solutions that you would never have thought of.

EXERCISE 27: *DISCOVERING THE QUALITIES YOU NEED*
Exploring your more negative reactions to trees can also help you identify some of the qualities you need to get in touch with.

Do you find any of the trees unfriendly, or off-putting? Be as accurate as you can in working out what aspects of a tree displease you or are not what you expected.

What relevance does this have for you?
What is it about this tree that touches things in yourself you find hard to acknowledge?
What memories does it stir up of problems that you have had in other contexts?

What quality would help you to move beyond this?
Where in this wood could you discover the quality you are in need of?
Focusing on this quality, let yourself be guided toward it in a walking meditation (Exercise 10, page 64).

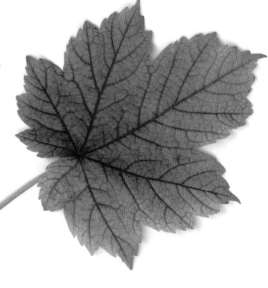

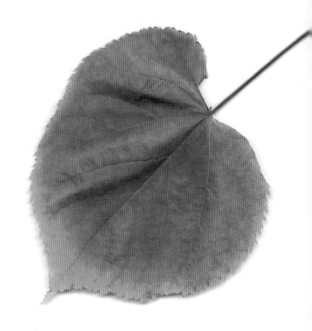

EXERCISE 28:
FINDING A NEW PERSPECTIVE

Identifying the qualities that you need to overcome a problem will guide you to a tree that can help you.

❶ What state are you in when you think about the problem?
Anxious, despairing, exhausted, in a hurry, angry, fearful, ...

❷ What state would you like to be in?
Confident, serene, full of energy, open, optimistic, ...

❸ Find a tree that holds the quality you identified in stage 2. Settle yourself there comfortably and let this quality soak into you, noticing any physical responses you may have to it.

❹ Bring your problem to mind again, holding your awareness of this quality at the same time.

Don't focus only on finding an answer; simply hold the presence of this quality (the physical responses you noticed in stage 3 will help you do this). When you least expect it the processes that are working on the subtle levels will lead you toward a new standpoint, from which you can envisage a new outcome.

EXERCISE 29:
ASKING A TREE A QUESTION

Follow these steps to discover the solutions the forest can offer.

❶ Formulate a question that encapsulates your problem, reflecting its most important aspects.

❷ With this question in mind, let yourself be led toward a tree in a walking meditation (Exercise 10, page 64).

❸ Settle yourself comfortably near this tree.

❹ Close your eyes and listen to what is happening inside you.

❺ Open your eyes and look at everything around you in detail, to bring your awareness into the present. Some hints of an answer to your question will be there - either an inner certainty, a sign, a symbol, or some feature near you that you realize mirrors your inner situation.

Don't worry if nothing comes immediately; it may take a little while.

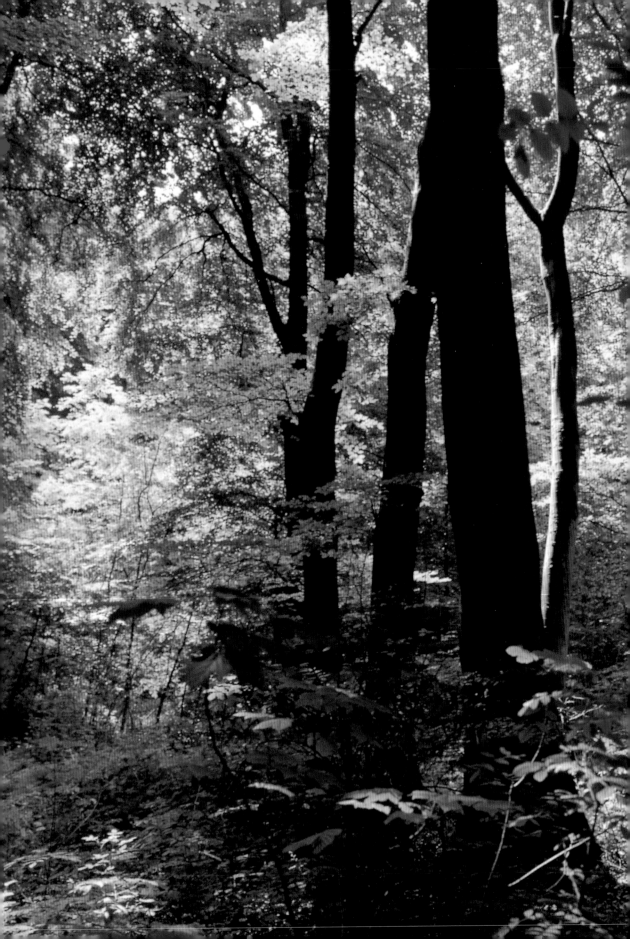

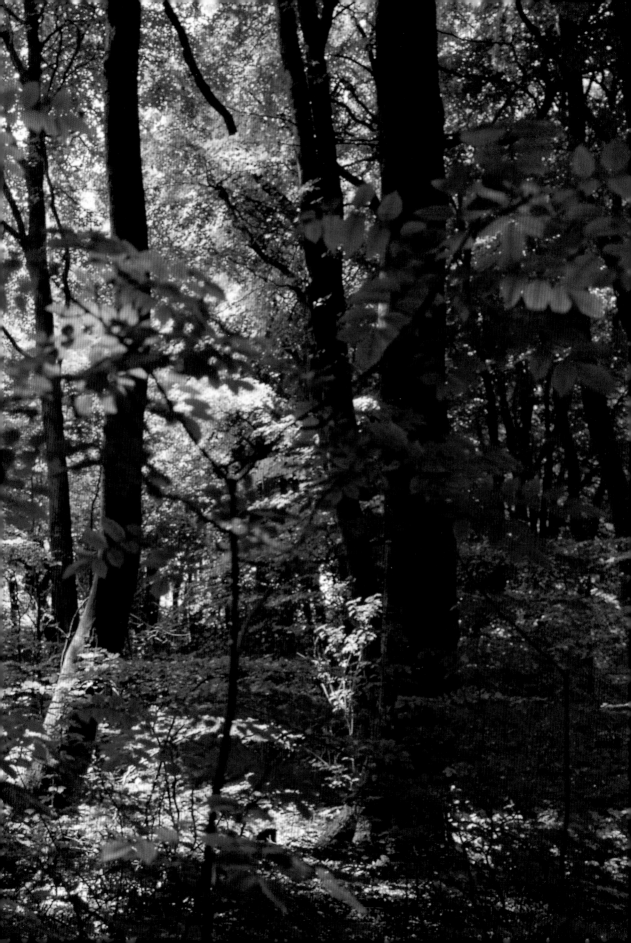

Tuning into tree qualities

Once you have found the tree you need to work with, go to meet it, following steps 2 and 3 of Exercise 11 (page 65). Sit comfortably underneath it and relax, opening yourself to the experience. When you feel ready, use breathing, sound, and movement (Exercises 18–20, pages 75–6) to tune into the tree and put yourself in resonance with it.

The qualities of the tree you are working with are not completely missing in you. We all have within us at some level the qualities of serenity, fluidity, autonomy, etc that we need, whether they are latent, or plain for all to see. As your energy field adapts to that of the tree, a common energy field is created. Here contact takes place between you and information is exchanged, enabling you to sense the quality present in the tree and to find it also in yourself.

When you work through the breathing, movement, and sound exercises your mental habits and your will may prevent you from being truly open to the experience and deceive you with false results. There is a fine line between hoping that something new will happen and subconsciously making a deliberate change. You might think that you are responding to the tree when in fact your response is something your mind has invented.

To make the most of these powerful exercises, check what you are doing frequently by asking yourself: "What part is my ordinary thinking and my will playing in this moment?" Such questioning will help you to understand yourself better and loosen the hold of your mental habits, so that eventually you will be able to recognize when you are inventing, making yourself more open for the true experience. The more you free yourself from the control of these old habits, the more space you create for your true nature and your higher self to express themselves through your energy bodies, thus creating a richer interaction with the tree.

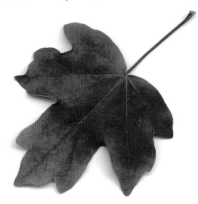

Continuing the process

A day spent in the woods may bring you a rich harvest of discoveries and understanding about yourself as well as about the trees you have been working with. But the experience doesn't stop there: it will go on working inside you and in your daily life for some time afterward. To maximize these continuing effects you should make time to recall and reflect upon your experiences when you are at home again. You can prepare for this in advance, by choosing something to bring back home with you from the tree that will remind you of your experience and the qualities of the tree. This symbol may be a part of the tree, a scrap of bark, a seed head, or a leaf, or something else that reminds you of that place, such as a stone you noticed. It could also be a photograph or sketch that captures something of the place, a recording of the sounds, or a mental reminder such as an image or word that came to you while you were there. Exercise 30 shows you how to use your symbol to connect again with the place and your experience.

When you leave the tree, whether you take something physical such as a twig or leaf, or a mental image, an emotion, or a sketch, remember to thank the tree for what it has given you.

EXERCISE 30:
RECONNECTING WITH THE QUALITY
To get back in touch with the experience you had with a tree, use your tree symbol or memento as a focal point.

Find a comfortable place where you will not be disturbed and relax deeply.
Let the atmosphere of that place and time re-create itself around you, as you see again what the place looks like, as you hear the sounds and smell the fragrances, as you recall the things you touched and the feelings that came to you.

Notice your breathing, its rhythm and pattern, and then take time to acknowledge how you feel now and what quality you are connected with.

Use this place you are in now as a new viewpoint from which to think again about a problem, or simply gain pleasure and refreshment from it.

The benefits from the experience

What you gain from an exchange with a tree depends on how ready you are to receive the energy message of its quality, and at what level you are ready to accept it and let change happen. The acceptance and response can occur at three levels.

Changes at the first level concern mostly the physical body, and occur very quickly. Perhaps your back ache or indigestion pains disappear after a few moments sitting against a tree. Such an experience is one of the most surprising and can seem almost magic. It can even occur when you do not have any expectation or preconceived ideas about what will happen.

The second level of response is emotional. Maybe you are in a state of confusion, but after an hour or so sitting against a tree the situation that seemed such a tangle suddenly unravels itself and you can see things more clearly.

The third level affects the deeper levels of consciousness. The contact with the tree's qualities gives you a new impetus and strength to deal with the areas where your life energy has got stuck. After such an experience you may feel that a reaction has been set off inside you, but you are not sure what it is. However a few days later you may find yourself in a familiar but difficult situation, and be surprised to notice that you are reacting in a new way, though you may not realize that this is the result of the inner process of change (see Case study, left).

When you are aware that some change is occurring at a deep level, even if you are not sure what it is, let the new energies find their way without too much pressure. Give yourself time to rest, since the early stages of the process can make you feel tired.

CASE STUDY

Monique, a therapist, prescribed the walnut oil for one of her clients, who knew nothing about the qualities of the tree oils. After a month of treatment the client reported that she had not felt anything special, but had kept on applying the oil daily anyway. During the month she had taken some important decisions, including giving up her career in accountancy, which she felt her father had pushed her into, and arranging to train as a social worker instead, which she had always wanted to do.

When Monique showed her the description of the walnut's quality of autonomy (see page 124), the client was stunned, since she had embarked on this major change without having any idea that there was a connection with the qualities embodied in the oil.

Dealing with feelings that arise

Some experiences triggered by working with tree energies may have a profound impact on your psyche. You may find yourself in an inner turmoil that seems overwhelming and impossible to cope with. Dealing with such feelings will be easier if you are prepared beforehand. Keep in mind that change is not a smooth linear process: it is more accurately represented as a spiral (see page 55), with a "jump" to a new level as transformation occurs. Periods of emotional chaos indicate a real process of transformation is taking place. It is in the cracks that we allow to appear in our old inner structures that the seeds of the new can plant themselves. If you tend to face your problems in the style of the "farmer" or "biologist" and you begin to shift toward the "shaman" or "mystic", you may feel disoriented for a while. But then you will begin to enjoy the wider view and the deeper understanding you have reached. The attitudes to nature and to illness outlined on pages 34-5 and 40-41 are landmarks along the way and will help you to understand where you are in the process.

During contact with a tree you set up a shared energy field where an exchange of information takes place. Thus any experiences you have are a part of you – they are not the result of an outside force imposing upon you, but a part of your inner life process. Therefore there is no point in fighting against any part of the experience; by acknowledging what is happening within, you can accept and integrate it. Trust in your own powers of transformation, helping them by relaxing and allowing yourself some peace and quiet. Also, listen to your energy bodies (Exercise 3, page 46) and your breathing. Soon you will realize that a new order is being created and a new inner peace is being born.

Some of your experiences among trees may seem fantastic. You may see colours or shapes or symbols, even hear voices, or suddenly feel that you are at one with the forest and linked to the whole of the universe. Welcome such experiences with pleasure, neither pushing them away in fear nor trying to make them stay. Consider in what way they have deepened your understanding of nature, of yourself, and of life, and what they mean for you at this moment. Remember that no two experiences with trees are the same (page 74) so if you share the experience with someone else, it will not have the same significance for them.

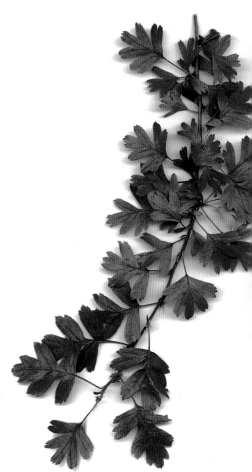

Supporting the healing process

The different qualities of the nine trees described in Chapter 4 are each helpful at different stages of the healing process, as shown in the table below.

   To find a tree to help you with a specific problem, use the description of the seven stages (pages 56-60) to help you decide which stage you have reached. From the table identify the qualities that would be beneficial to you at this stage. If the given tree that manifests this quality is not available in your area, use Exercises 24 and 26 (pages 84 and 133) to find a tree with the quality you need.

STAGES OF THE HEALING PROCESS	REACTION
❶ The problem appears	I am shocked, hurt, knocked off balance, forced to re-evaluate
❷ The ego resists	I blame someone else or some external factor
❸ Seeing what the problem reveals	My mind finds a strategy to limit my suffering
❹ Experimenting with another attitude	I identify behaviour that I could change, and try out a new attitude
❺ New qualities come in	The new behaviour has become part of me. I see the problem more objectively
❻ The new attitude changes the situation	The new situation gives me more inner freedom
❼ I integrate what has happened	I am reborn, but need to take care that I do not slip back into old ways of behaving

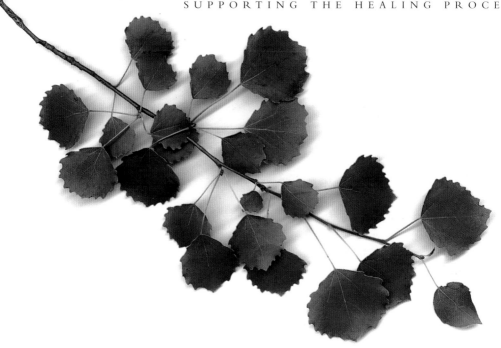

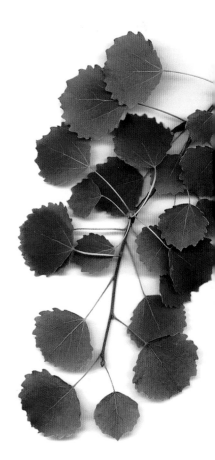

RELEVANT TREE   BENEFICIAL QUALITIES

Relevant tree	Beneficial qualities
Beech	Serenity, confidence
Fir	Fluidity
Birch	Gentleness, reconciliation
Hawthorn	Alignment
Fir	Fluidity
Box	Liberation
Broom	Renewal, rebirth
Walnut	Autonomy, responsibility
Box	Continuity, liberation
Fir	Fluidity
Hawthorn	Alignment
Wild rose	Openness
Pine	Light, vitality
Pine	Light, vitality
Walnut	Autonomy, responsibility
Box	Continuity, liberation
Wild rose	Openness
Broom	Renewal, rebirth

Facilitating a change of viewpoint

When faced with a problem we tend to have a fixed set of responses and follow a familiar pattern of thought to find a solution. Focusing on the problem during a walk in the forest, or working through any of the exercises with trees, can help to bring about a new perception of the problem, enabling us to find more creative solutions. This change of attitude may be triggered in one of four different ways.

Contact with the living reality of the tree

In the midst of the forest the feeling of being linked with the whole web of life can come upon you with surprising suddenness. The trees in their deep-rooted silence, that seem to be watching and aware, are fully alive and powerfully present. Experiencing this for the first time may feel like a threat and set off the defence mechanisms we deploy to resist the force of life. But once you get used to this sense of presence you can enjoy it, because it puts you in touch with what unites us all, the sense of the life force within.

An experience of this force can revolutionize your understanding of life itself, as well as your attitude to a problem, but it will not happen to order or from trying. It can come while doing any of the exercises of this book, or when you are just resting for a moment sitting against a tree. However it is more likely to occur when your mind is not stuck in habitual thinking patterns. Exercise 7 on page 57 helps you free your mind from superfluous thoughts.

Revelation

When you ask a tree a question (Exercise 29, page 135), as in any contact with a tree, a shared energy field is set up between you and the tree. Sometimes an exchange of energy brings about a temporary energy shift in you, changing your usual patterns of thinking. This makes way for new ideas and a new perspective on the problem, and often brings new inspiration for solving it.

The living metaphor

When you set off into the woods with a problem in mind, the situations or objects you encounter can take on a special significance. For example you may find a patch of brambles blocking your way and be so determined to stick to the path you have chosen that you struggle on, trying to force a way through. When you find that impossible you turn back in fury and frustration at your failure, and collapse exhausted on to a nearby log. From this new viewpoint you notice another path, much easier and more direct, that you were blinded to by your earlier determination.

In the same way, your problem may have a simple solution that you have not been able to see because you are so determined to do things in your usual way. Perhaps a solution will turn up if you relax a little and stay open to what life brings you. This may sound a bit simplistic, but when you live through it and discover this connection for yourself, it can be a revelation that changes everything. Sometimes no such insight presents itself, and this too may be significant.

Understanding in the context of the forest

Often a particular feature of the forest will have a relevance to you. For example, a mass of brambles and undergrowth can be taken to represent your life problems. Working with a partner as in the blind person and their guardian angel (Exercise 15, page 69), you can attempt to get through this obstacle blindfolded. Your partner should watch and tell you afterward what they observed about how you tackled the task. This will have parallels with the way you tackle a problem in real life and so can give you insights into different ways of approaching it.

The tree as a therapeutic mirror

In a consultation with a therapist, as in the meeting with any other person, a shared energy field is set up, where each person's energy shifts to adapt to the other. A therapist will consider the patient's problems from his or her own level of consciousness, and each new incident in the session, such as a question that sets off more feelings, or goes into another aspect of the problem, changes the energy state of one or both, thus resulting in a shift of the combined energy field. Exercise 31 gives you practice in noticing these shifts.

A tree does not have the shifting feelings, thoughts, and soul state of a therapist. Whereas in the contact with a therapist the balance is maintained by adjustments on both sides, in the contact with the tree it is only the patient that adjusts. The tree is a constant; it cannot be influenced, so the patient is inevitably brought back to themselves. In this meeting with a tree its energy stirs a response in us; we may stay with it and allow its quality to resonate and increase within us, or, if we feel it is too much, we may choose to resist this meeting with ourselves.

Whatever response the contact with the tree triggers, the experience will always enlarge our field of awareness. The power of the tree carries us to another plane, where human patterns of behaviour are no longer in force. Our consciousness expands and our view of reality changes as we look at the world and our own problems with new eyes. At the same time we get to know ourselves better, since to recognize the life force in a tree we have to recognize it in ourselves. This discovery in ourselves puts us in even stronger resonance with the tree.

EXERCISE 31: *NOTICING INNER CHANGE*
This exercise will give you practice in noticing the changes that occur as you approach a tree, and as your energy field adapts to that of the tree.

Choose a tree from those around you and make a visual contact. Notice what is going on inside you as you do so.
Move half the distance toward the tree, stop and note again what is happening within. Come close to the tree. What has changed?

When you have done this exercise a few times you will find yourself becoming more aware of how you adapt to other people. You will also develop a greater awaresness of what is going on in your inner world and in your body, which won't then have to come up with all sorts of symptoms in order to get your attention.

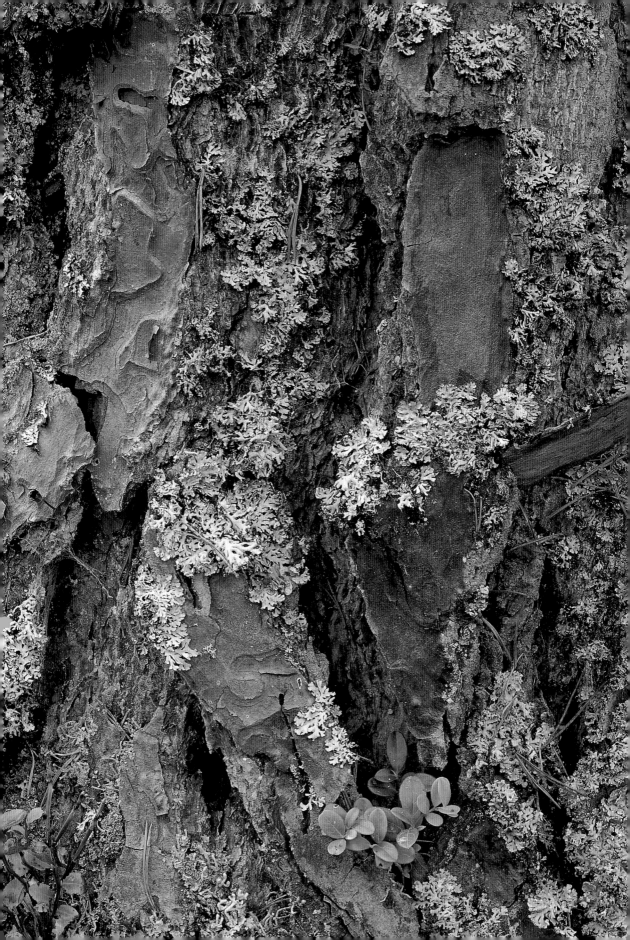

Fundamental tasks

Followed in the order given, these nine steps will help you resolve a crisis or problem by developing the qualities you need, rather than by searching for a fixed solution. Each step is best supported by a particular tree energy, as described below.

❶ BECOMING RELAXED
This is the first step - otherwise the energies of stress will lead to aggression and struggle, and will never step aside to let your higher self play its part. Open yourself to the peace of the forest. *The fir energy encourages the fluidity and letting go necessary for relaxation.*

❾ MOTIVATING YOURSELF
Once you have made a decision you need to take responsibility for it and then take action.
The walnut provides the energy of autonomy to help in this.

❽ MAKING A DECISION
A true life decision should honour the things that really matter to you and deepen your respect for who you really are. The intimacy of the forest provides a place where we can re-centre ourselves - a prerequisite for making any serious decision.
The energies of hawthorn also facilitate this centring process.

❼ MAKING A NEW START
The only stable foundation for the future is a past that has been accepted and integrated - old patterns disentangled and old wounds healed. Whatever happened in the past, we can thank it for bringing us to the place we have now reached. New growth in the forest and on individual trees reminds us that the life force is unstoppable and can inspire your own new start.
Broom provides the special energy of renewal.

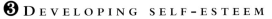

❷ SEEING MORE CLEARLY

Once you are relaxed you can begin to see the realities of the problem more clearly.

The energy of pine brings light to bear on a problem and makes it easier to understand.

❸ DEVELOPING SELF-ESTEEM

It is essential to learn to love yourself, because only in the depth of your own heart can you find unconditional love. How much you can love life and other people will be limited if there is a limit on how much you love yourself.

The birch, embodying gentleness that is not weak or sentimental, helps your self-esteem to grow.

❹ IMPROVING COMMUNICATION

Before you can learn to be open with others, you need to clear the channels of communication within yourself, allowing your true self to express itself. As a catalyst for this process, sit in a woodland clearing and focus on the contrast between the open space and its boundaries, using Exercise 12 on page 67.

The energies of wild rose are a support in any process of opening.

❺ BUILDING SELF-CONFIDENCE

This involves getting in touch with your inner strength, which you can count on in any situation.

In a forest there are many images of strength, some more genuine than others. Learning to differentiate between them is good practice for detecting any false note in your own self-assurance.

The beech embodies true self-confidence and inner strength.

❻ BECOMING FREE OF THE PAST

The wounds we have suffered, whether or not we have a conscious memory of them, need to come to the surface to be faced and healed.

Some places in a forest have a magical power to put us in touch with the depths of our being; in such a place you will feel very small in relation to the power that is present.

The energies of box will help you find release from the past through facing past hurts.

What trees can heal in us

The exercises in this chapter and Chapter 3 present techniques for meeting and working with trees and their healing energies. But it is not always necessary to get into profound contact with a tree to benefit from its healing energies. Being among trees for the pleasure of it can also be healing on the physical, emotional, mental, and spiritual levels.

Take a walk in the woods and let yourself enjoy each moment, each detail, in its simplicity; breathe in the atmosphere. Give yourself the freedom to find a comfortable place to sit, and enjoy. Being able to make the most of the good things life offers us is just as important as being able to look deeply and honestly into our inner processes.

PHYSICAL LEVEL
RECONNECTING WITH YOUR BODY
When you spend time in the forest in full awareness, as in the walking meditation (Exercise 10, page 64), your gestures and movements stop being automatic and lead you to become more present. Even the simple act of finding how to sit comfortably against a tree makes you more aware of your physical sensations and possible tensions, and through this you reconnect yourself and rediscover how you are living in your body.

RELEASING TENSION
A walk in the forest is in itself relaxing, and thus helps reveal and release some of the tight spots in the body which hinder it from working as well as it could. Being in the presence of trees such as fir, which embody a quality of fluidity, can help to release such tensions. Different systems are affected in different people, but freer breathing, better elimination, and better sleep, as well as a lifting away of stress and persistent fatigue, can all result.

REGAINING CONFIDENCE IN YOUR BODY
When you feel more present in your body and your breathing and your other systems are working better, you will feel more confidence in your physical abilities. As you explore the forest you may find yourself abandoning any limits you have set on your way of moving, as you climb over fallen trees and overcome other obstacles. The limits we assume to be an inevitable part of growing old are only a mental barrier, which can be dissolved through contact with the energy of a tree. After such an experience you will return home invigorated and with fresh confidence in your physical capacities and yourself.

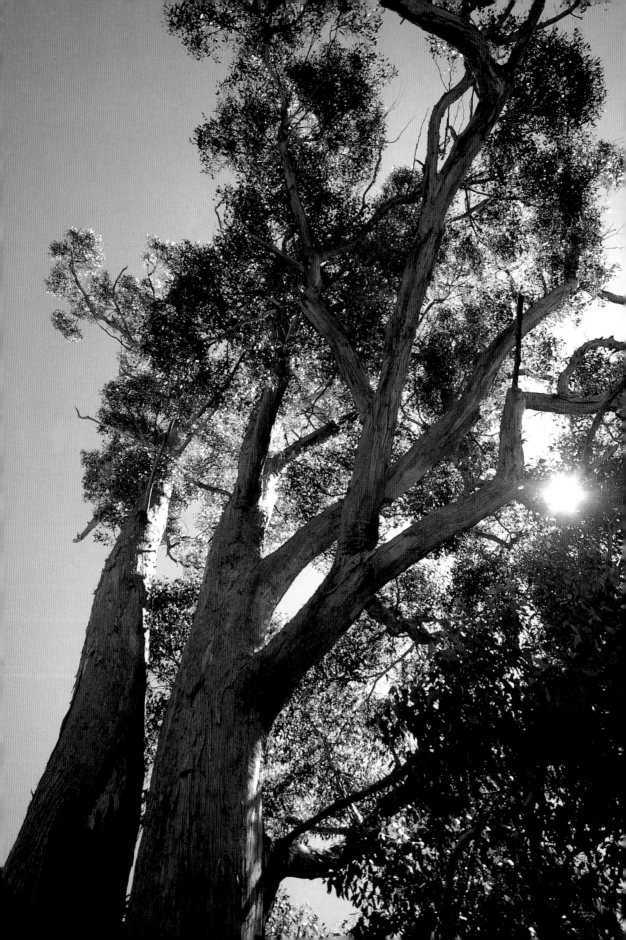

EMOTIONAL LEVEL
RELEASING PERSONAL AND ARCHETYPAL FEARS

The forest can inspire fear, an echo from ancient race memories that may be made more potent by the sense that the depths of the forest represent the depths of the unconscious. On the surface it translates into fear of getting lost and the fear of encountering danger. To overcome such fears, start at the edge of the forest and look for a tree that you find reassuring. Walk over to it and focus on your fear, staying at the foot of the tree and breathing calmly until you feel again the reassuring qualities that attracted you to it. When your confidence has returned, repeat the process with another tree, deeper in the forest. In this way you can journey into the heart of the forest via these landmarks of confidence. At each tree, look back and make sure you can recognize where you came from, so you can follow the same path with trust on your return journey.

LEARNING TO LIVE IN THE PRESENT

A walk in the woods is a good place to practise being in the present, which is necessary if you want to learn and enjoy all you can in your surroundings. You may set off full of preconceptions about the world around you, but you will soon be brought back to reality when you find yourself caught in the brambles, or notice that where you have chosen to sit and contemplate is an anthill.

REDISCOVERING YOUR INNER CHILD

Take a cue from the way children play when they are in the woods, and let your inner child rediscover the delight of being spontaneous and free from your usual restraints.

MENTAL LEVEL
ENLARGING YOUR FIELD OF PERCEPTION

The exercises on extending your five senses (Exercises 12-17, Chapter 3) show you how much more you can perceive if you give yourself the freedom to do so. This wider vision enables you to find new perspectives on situations that concern you.

In the forest all is calm and most of the mind's activity arises from the mind itself. Releasing your mind from superfluous thoughts (Exercise 7, page 57) and directing it toward this calm, will allow you to relax into a state of peace and wellbeing.

THE TRAPS OF THE MIND

Your mind governs how you experience the world, since you evaluate events according to beliefs that are part of your culture, your education, or "common sense". We see only a glimmer of these beliefs in the conscious mind, while the rest lurks hidden in the unconscious. In the forest, without the usual distractions, it is easier to detect these determining notions and recognize the distortions in your self-image.

SPIRITUAL LEVEL
EXPERIENCING THE LIFE FORCE
Contact with trees offers us a direct connection to the essence of life. The forest, in its spendour and its power, enshrines something that is greater than ourselves, beyond structured belief systems and day-to-day concerns. This opens up the spiritual dimension that is a living presence, already and eternally there within us.

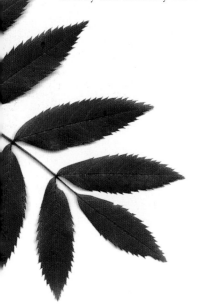

MAKING THE LINK WITH LIFE
In the forest, all that you see is part of the cycle of life, and you gradually come closer to discovering what is truly alive in yourself, your essence. The aliveness of nature raises an echo from that aliveness in yourself, in a spiritual experience that connects you with the life force.

The trees that are all around us have a tremendous potential to help and heal us. With an understanding of how our crises and problems arise and are resolved, we can find ways of using their energies in our healing. Close observation of a tree's physical form reveals its most evident qualities, but by cultivating our intuition and refining our senses we can discover so much more. The trees of the forest hold out to us a helping hand, but they also challenge us to become more responsible for our own self-development: "Come to meet us so that you can evolve further - but first evolve further so that we can meet." The techniques presented in this book guide you on the first steps of your journey to a true meeting with trees.

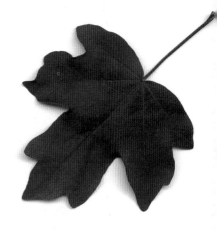

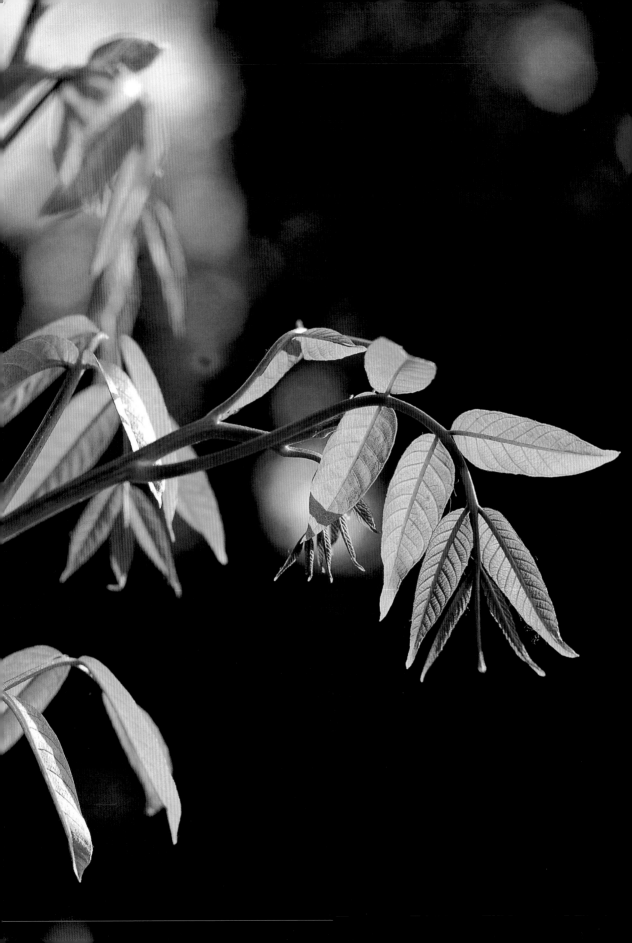

Afterword

The living approach to trees presented in this book can be used to great benefit within the domains of teaching, personal development, and therapy, and wherever there is a need to be creative in finding new solutions to the problems that face us.

Such "intelligent" contact with our natural environment requires learning through direct experience and apprenticeship. Used in the teaching of other disciplines, these approaches could give children the tools they need to build their own knowledge and reveal their gifts that often are undeveloped in the academic system. Such a style of learning encourages the delight of discovery and encourages the learner to go further, since what they are finding out is really alive. Thus children can get in touch with the life force within themselves and discover their links with the rest of nature. It is through this discovery that they learn a respect for life - for their own, for other people, and for the natural world. They also come to see that reality has many facets, and thus they can come to respect others' views and refine their sense of judgement without becoming critical.

There are many ways in which the creativity inspired by nature can be applied and enjoyed in our lives, and if you set out on this path you will find many more for yourself and for the people and situations you are involved with. What this book offers is not another system of fixed ideas or prescribed solutions, but a set of tools which can help you construct new models of thinking which in turn create new attitudes.

I feel that humanity is on the threshold of discovering a completely new level of reality. The seeds of potential are beginning to grow within each of us and will bring about true change in the world as they begin to flower. It is my hope that creative contact with the wonders of nature will help these seeds grow and flourish.

Resources

Dictionnaire des symbols, Robert Lafont, Paris, 1969

Flore forestière Francaise tome 1, Idf edition (Ministère de l'Agriculture Français), Paris 1989

Brahma Kumaris World Spiritual University Staff, ed., *Visions of a Better World,* Brahma Kumaris World Spiritual University, New York, 1993

Bross, Jacques, *Les arbres de France,* Plon, 1987

Chase, Pamela Louise and Pawlik, Jonathan, *Trees for Healing,* Newcastle Publishing Co Inc, California, 1991

Coats, Callum, *Living Energies,* Gateway Books, Bath, 1996

Cook, Roger, *The Tree of Life,* Thames and Hudson, New York, 1995

Gimbel, Theo, *Healing with Color and Light,* Simon and Schuster, New York, 1994

Honervogt, Tanmaya, *The Power of Reiki,* An Owl Book, Henry Holt and Company, New York, 1998

Langer, Ellen, *Mindfulness,* Addison-Wesley, Reading, Massachussetts, 1989

McLean, Dorothy, *To Honor the Earth,* HarperSan Francisco, 1991

Mees, Dr L F C, *La maladie ... une bénédiction,* Les Trois Arches, Chatou, 1987

Mendelsohn, Robert, *How to Raise a Healthy Child ... in Spite of your Doctor,* Ballantine Books, New York, 1987

Milner, J Edward, *The Tree Book,* Trafalgar Square, North Pomfret, Vermont, 1994

Mindell, Arnold, *Dreambody,* Sigo Press, Boston, 1982

Paterson, Jacqueline Memory, *Tree Wisdom,* Thorsons, San Francisco, 1996

Pearce, Fred, *Turning up the Heat: Our Perilous Future in the Global Greenhouse,* Bodley Head, London, 1989

Popcorn, Faith and Marigold Lys, *Clicking,* HarperCollins, New York, 1996

Pribram, *Synchronicity,* Bantam Books, New York, 1987

Purce, Jill, *The Mystic Spiral,* Thames and Hudson, New York, 1990

Sheldrake, Rupert, *Seven Experiments that Could Change the World,* Berkley Publishing Group, New York, 1996

—*The Rebirth of Nature,* Bantam Books, Inner Traditions International, Rochester, Vermont, 1994

Vogt, Nathalie and Michel, *La Foret du Rhin secrète et légendaire,* published by the authors, 1995

Photographic credits

p 2, 6-7, 8-9, Alan Watson/Forest Light (FL); p 10-11 David Woodfall/Woodfall Wild Images (WWI); p 13, 14-5, 16 Alan Watson/FL; p 17 Maurizio Biancarelli/WWI; p 21 Ronald Sheridan/Ancient Art and Architecture; p 22-3 *background image:* Science Photo Library; p 22 Alan Watson/FL; p 23 *from top:* Alan Watson/FL, Gaia Books, Steve Austin/WWI, Biophoto Associates/SPL; p 26-7 Steve Teague; p 31 Rob Blakers/WWI; p 34-5, 36-7 Alan Watson/FL; p 38 Kathy Collins/WWI; p 39 David Woodfall/WWI; p 40-41 Deni Bown; p 47 John MacPherson/WWI; p 50, 52-3 Alan Watson/FL; p 57, 58 Gaia Books; p 59 Bob Gibbons/WWI; p 61 Gaia Books; p 62 Mark Hamblin/WWI; p 63, 64-5 Maurizio Biancarelli/WWI; p 67, 71 Alan Watson/FL; p 72-3 Kathy Collins/WWI; p 74 Nigel Hicks/WWI; p 77 Alan Watson/FL; p 80-1 David Woodfall/WWI; p 82-3, 86 Alan Watson/FL; p 88 Deni Bown; p 89 David Woodfall/WWI; p 93 Patrice Bouchardon; p 94 Kathy Collins/WWI; p 95 Niall Benvie/Oxford Scientific Films (OSF); p 96 Deni Bown; p 97 Steve Austin/WWI; p 98 Maurizio Biancarelli/WWI; p 99 Alan Watson/FL; p 100 Hans Reinhard/OSF; p 101 Niall Benvie/OSF; p 102 Deni Bown/OSF; p 103 David Woodfall/WWI; p 104, p 105 *top:* Bob Gibbons/WWI; *bottom:* Deni Bown/OSF; p 106 Niall Benvie/OSF; p 107 Alan Watson/FL; p 108 William Paton/OSF; p 109 Alan Watson/FL; p 110, 111 David Woodfall/WWI; p 112 Deni Bown; p 113 *top:* Steve Austin/WWI; *bottom:* John Robinson/WWI; p 114 Steve Austin/WWI; p 115 David Woodfall/WWI; p 116 Deni Bown; p 118 Bob Gibbons/WWI; p 119 Steve Teague; p 120 Bob Gibbons/WWI; p 122 Alan Watson/FL; p 123 Steve Teague; p 124 Bob Gibbons/WWI; p 125 *top:* John Robinson/WWI; *bottom:* G I Bernard/OSF; p 126 Steve Austin/WWI; p 127 Michael Leach/OSF; p 128 Deni Bown; p 129 Bob Gibbons/WWI; p 130, 131 Alan Watson/FL; p 133-5, 139, 141, 143, 148-9, 152-3 Gaia Books; p 136-7 Steve Teague; p 147, 151 Alan Watson/FL; p 154 Steve Teague. Artwork on p 43 and p 44 by Mark Preston.

Publisher's acknowledgements

The publishers would like to thank: Anne Brabyn, Tamsin Juggins, Patrick O'Halloran, and Deborah Pate for editorial assistance and research; Helena Petre for proofreading; Jenny and Owen Dixon for help with photographic illustrations; and Lynn Bresler for proofreading and the index.

Index

If you liked *The Healing Energies of Trees,* you should read:

THE HEALING ENERGIES OF WATER
by Charlie Ryrie

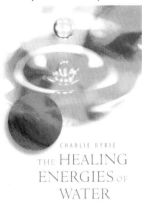

This book explores the human relationship with water throughout
the centuries, explains water's importance for the health of the
body, outlines different water remedies for a variety of ailments,
and, finally, suggests how to use energized water in the home
or garden for health, meditation, and relaxation.

ISBN 1-885203-72-1

THE DETOX PLAN
FOR BODY, MIND, AND SPIRIT
by Jane Alexander

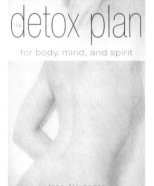

The Detox Plan is a clear, simple, and definitive
guide to ridding yourself of unwanted toxins,
clutter, and negative thoughts. It offers readers
easy, practical ways to integrate healthy living
into even the most hectic lifestyles.

ISBN 1-885203-70-5

For a complete catalog, call or write:
Tuttle Publishing/Journey Editions, RR1 Box 231-5, North Clarendon, VT 05759-9700
phone: (802) 773-8930 • fax: (802) 773-6993 • toll-free: (800) 526-2778

• •

9 healing oils ...
9 supporting audio cassettes ...
to help you accomplish 9 fundamental life tasks:

becoming relaxed: **Fir**

seeing more clearly
into the problem: **Pine**

developing self-esteem: **Birch**

improving communication
with yourself and others: **Wild rose**

building self-confidence: **Beech**

becoming free of the past: **Box**

making a new start: **Broom**

making a decision: **Hawthorn**

motivating yourself: **Walnut**

The cassettes offer you the chance to journey at your own
pace through this sequence of life tasks. Each step is
made easier by using the appropriate oil, which will
bring into your awareness the inner qualities
you need as you face your trials and
solve your problems, and support
you on your chosen path.

The cassettes and oils can be
ordered as a complete set or individually.

Available from:
Patrice Bouchardon, PO Box 99651, Troy, MI 48099-9651
or Lieve Bonne, Solsties, Ezelstraat 39, 8000 Brugge, Belgium
Tel/fax: 011 32 50 33 87 54

Also available from:
Gaia Books Ltd, 20 High Street, Stroud, Glos. GL5 1AZ, UK
Tel: 011 44 1453 752985 Fax: 011 44 1453 752987
email: Lyn@gaiabooks.co.uk

Patrice Bouchardon is available to run workshops and
seminars worldwide. Please contact Patrice c/o
Lieve Bonne in Belgium or Lyn Hemming at
Gaia Books Ltd. (see left for both addresses).